Sexuality and Motherhood

Irene Walton
M Sc, B Ed(Hons), RM, MTD, FETC, CMS

Books for Midwives Press
Books for Midwives Press is a joint publishing venture
between The Royal College of Midwives
and Haigh & Hochland Publications Ltd

Published by Books for Midwives Press, 174a Ashley Road, Hale, Cheshire, WA15 9SF, England

© 1994, Irene Walton

Reprinted 1995

First edition

ISBN 1-898507-07-4

British Library Cataloguing in Publication Data
A catalogue record for this book is available from the British Library

Printed in Great Britain by Cromwell Press Ltd

Acknowledgements

I would like to dedicate this book to my husband Alan who is truly 'the wind beneath my wings'.

I would also like to give my loving thanks to my daughter Jane, to my son Andrew and to my mother for their help, support, interest and encouragement. Amongst my band of family supporters who all deserve my appreciation, there are in particular Margaret and Alan Oldfield, who have unfailingly and humorously ensured that I kept to the task.

I would also like to express my appreciation and gratitude to Henry Hochland who made this book possible in so many ways.

Contents

PART ONE

Sexuality as a Construct

Introduction

So God created man in his own image, in the image of God he created him;
male and female he created them. And God blessed them, and God said to
them, "Be fruitful and multiply, and fill the earth..And God saw everything
that he had made, and behold it was very good.
Genesis Ch.1, v.26-31

Sexuality! So short a word and so powerful! Who can read it, say it or think it without evoking strong and mixed mental images. It permeates our very being and affects everything we do, everything we hold dear and everything we transmit as our physical and cultural heritage. Yet how many of us deny this aspect of humanity both in our own lives and in those of the people around us?

On entering the midwifery profession as a mature married student with two children I noticed immediately the lack of emphasis put on this part of life. Initially I was amused when I was taught that the function of the pelvic floor was to allow 'micturition, defecation and parturition'. What had happened to coition? I looked at the women in the clinical areas in awe as I hadn't realized there were so many virgin births . Previously I had thought there was only one - but I jest, and I shouldn't, for it became increasingly apparent to me that this oversight was not a joking matter.

We live our lives within a framework of rules and meanings which enable us socially to construct our reality and act rationally. However as Schultze (1953) says, because of this we come to the 'the conclusion that, "rational" action on the common sense level is always action within an unquestioned and undetermined frame of constructs of typicalities of the setting, the motives, the means and the ends, the courses of action and personalities involved and taken for granted.' So what does it mean if a part of human existence is rejected in an area where it cannot be denied? There are no simple answers, or if there are, I have not got them for you. It may be to do with the `invisibility and muting' (Dube, Leacock and Ardener, 1986) of women, i.e. a reflection of their apparent powerlessness and passivity in society. This gives rise to a contradiction in terms. How can a powerless group possess power? As they obviously cannot, but in fact do, then this power has to be denied. So the sexuality of women is denied and we see this in various ways. Does the nude model in a `girlie' magazine look like a sexual being or a passive object? Can the mother and child image convey anything other than the Madonna? By denying the sexuality of women, and mothers in particular, we make it something to ashamed of, or frightened about, so a `taboo' of silence is formulated. This silence is manifest through praxis.

It is broken up and refracted through all the symbols, rituals and social interactions of midwifery. For example it is well documented (Kirkham, 1989) that midwives infantilize the women in their care through the use of language, and children (notwithstanding Freud) are thought to be asexual beings in our culture.

My purpose in writing this book is to examine the concept of sexuality with all its wealth of meanings of emotion, gender and experience in order to reduce confusion and heighten awareness of its relevance in the lives of people of all ages. I particularly want to emphasize the importance of such intelligence to the understanding of women as mothers and sexual beings and in the development of midwifery as a holistic caring profession where midwives are truly 'with woman'.

CHAPTER ONE

In the Beginning

Well, not quite in the beginning and not everywhere

Female desire is crucial to our whole social structure. Small wonder it is so closely obscured, so endlessly pursued, so frequently recast and reformulated.
Rosalind Coward (1984)

Sexuality, what is it? Is it embedded in nature? Is it the representation of a powerful, overwhelming force that must be fought over and controlled by the moral, religious or medical guardians of society and their opponents. Or is it a socially constructed phenomenon which is only meaningful in the cultural and temporal context of the discourse? These are questions that may never be able to be answered fully, but what is certain is that sexuality is not confined to an individual's private feelings, practices, and commitments. Nor is it simply about pleasure and pain, eroticism and fulfilment, or even fear and loathing. It belongs in the social arena. It is in the full glare of the public gaze and brings together in one concept the diverse meanings of a culture, those of beliefs, values, traditions, power and social hierarchies. As Foucault (1979) says:

Sexuality must not be thought of as a kind of natural given which power tries to hold in check, or as an obscure domain which knowledge tries gradually to uncover. It is the name that can be given to a historical construct.

So to understand sexuality in a modern Western context it is necessary to look at some of the ways that sexuality was viewed in the past and the cycles that recur, for history is not necessarily the story of a linear progression towards advancement. It is extremely difficult to present an unbiased, objective picture of sexuality through the ages and impossible to say what it was for women and for mothers in particular until relatively recently. Most men and nearly all women could not write, so history is delivered throught he eyes of a small section of society. The sexuality of women as mothers can only be glimpsed obliquely through reference to the times in general.

All of us, all our lives have been taught to make judgements based on the current culture and prevailing morals. These judgements are based on our deepest emotions and form the present values and social norms. So it is extremely difficult to look at history from a post-enlightenment perspective and shed the clear light of truth (if there is such a thing) upon it. At best we can only get a flavour, but a necessary flavour, if we wish to understand the sexual customs, values and codes of today. There is also another consideration to be taken into account, that of idealism and reality. People's behaviour in reality very often differs quite markedly from the idealized social behaviour as exemplified in the literature or religious teachings of the day and so the past must be approached with scepticism.

Freud would have had a field day with the neuroses, delusions, hallucinations and hysteria thrown up by the repression of sexuality over the last 2,000 years. In the first 500 or so years A.D. there was a free attitude to sexuality that over the remaining 1,500 years has become more and more repressed. This is not to say that it was not surrounded by social mores, just as any social process is, rather that there was a healthier attitude. Sex was seen as part of everyday life, a pleasure and a joy for all. Marriage was looser and women were freer. It was not an immoral time in itself, it just did not profess a Christian concept of morality. Women were free to take lovers both before and after marriage and men were free to chase any woman. In fact they could seduce lower rank women with relative impunity and, although not able to take a higher rank woman against her will in the normal course of events, he could win her hand (and body) in contest. Virginity and sexual continence were not prized virtues. In many of the early folk tales the hero is given the king's daughter as a prize for deeds well done. It is only in later or Christianized versions that he is given her hand in marriage. Although in many respects women were treated as chattels in sexual matters they were relatively free and were not required to be passive. They could do, and often did do, the running in the mating game. This being so they were probably more able to take the initiative in bed as well than they were in later ages. There is very little extant literature from the Celts of this time, except from the Irish and it is clear from their writings (Rattray Taylor, 1953) that there were few inhibitions about sex and sexuality. For example, when Princess Findabair mentions to her mother that she fancies the messenger from the enemy camp, her mother suggests that she sleeps with him that night. Marriage for the Celts was a temporary and pragmatic affair, and to be a bastard was a mark of honour rather than disgrace. It meant that a valiant knight had slept with one's mother. This pride in bastardy continued for hundreds of years and to some extent into the present century. William the Conqueror, King Arthur and Charlemagne were reputed to be bastards almost as if it was a requirement for a hero. At this time marriage was civil contract. It was not conducted by a priest and did not take place in Church. It could be made by simply making a declaration to each other, witnesses were useful but not necessary, and this 'spousal' constituted a legitimate marriage. However this was soon to end.

In 786 A.D. the Anglo Saxon Synod decreed,

> that the son of a meretricious union shall be debarred from legally inheriting.... We command, then, in order to avoid fornication that every layman shall have one legitimate wife, and every woman shall have one legitimate husband, in order that they may have and beget legitimate heirs according to God's law.(Rattray Taylor, 1953)

Now not only was sexuality to be bound, it was to be gender, legally and religiously bound. St Paul's first letter to the Corinthians (6,9-10) and his letter to Timothy (1,9-10) condemning adulterers, sexual perverts, immoral persons and sodomites saw to that. Now not only were there sins but there were sins of the flesh and they were categorized into four ascending subgroups. The first consisted of those who prostituted themselves. In the second were those who committed adultery, those who seduced other men's wives and those wives who allowed themselves to be seduced. The third were 'mollities' (Aries, 1985) a derogatory word used to describe people who were passive (or used practices to prolong or delay the climax) who were not in fact, as the macho Romans liked men to be, virile and aggressive: The fourth was also something derived from the Roman culture, the 'masculorum concubitores' men who go to bed together. Lesbians did not tend to figure in the sinning category, probably because women did not figure highly in Paulian thinking except as the channel for sin to enter the world, and so women and their sexuality was ignored. The outcome was that now there were new sins in the world, the sins of the flesh, and included amongst them were homosexuality, which until then had been widely practised especially in the Hellenic world, and had been considered normal. There was also the new ideal of virginity for both women and men, and moreover within as well as without marriage. However, although Paul was not too bothered with procreation, because for him the Kingdom of Heaven was at hand, he thought that if desires could not be controlled they had better be satisfied within marriage, and so began the new sexual system of Christendom.

As Jean-Louis Flandrin (1985) observes:

> A basic tenet of Christian morality is an overwhelming disapproval of the pleasures of the flesh, because it trammels up the soul in the body, preventing it from aspiring towards God. We must eat to live but we must be careful not to enjoy the pleasures of the table too much. We are obliged to embrace the opposite sex in order to produce children, but we should not get too fond of the pleasures of sex. Sexuality was given for the purpose of reproduction. We abuse it if we use it for other ends, such as pleasure.

This was taken to such extremes that most of the Church's teachers held that husbands and wives who had intercourse for pleasure were committing a mortal sin. For those who could not refrain there was a garment specially recommended to reduce contact and pleasure. This was a heavy nightshirt, the 'chemise cagoule' with a hole in the front through which the process of impregnation could take place. This attitude to marriage is still to some extent in existence, although in the Alternative Prayer Book of the Church of England 1980 the priest does say at the commencement of the marriage service that:

It is given, that with delight and tenderness they may know each other in love, and through the joy of their bodily union, may strengthen the union of their hearts and lives.

Marriage was a contract and represented the handing over of a woman's fertility as part of a paid agreement. A woman's wants and desires did not figure at all. Marriage enabled perpetuation of 'blood' and inheritance by peaceful settlement rather than by force or abduction. The rites associated with this are still part of the wedding ceremonies of today; the handing over or giving away of the bride, and the representation of the bride's claim to the man's estate - the giving of a ring by the bridegroom. Marriage was not about love, it was about power and social stability. It regulated men's sexual desires and it consolidated the family wealth. This led to a proliferation of marriage between cousins when there was an amount of wealth within the family. It reunited, consolidated and enhanced the family holdings. Although there was now disapproval of abduction as a means of achieving a bride and wealth, there was still heavy reliance on patrimony and exploitation. This led to incestuous marriage which the Church had defined as within the seventh degree. This was not abolished until the Council of Rome of 1059 (Duby, 1978). Marriage in this case transformed a young man's life. He now became a man of property and was able to set up himself with a new household. But this was only true for the eldest son in the household. The younger sons did not have much of a chance of having a bride so they resorted to wandering and freely availing themselves of peasant women and servant girls, widows and 'maidens' who freely gave their favours. Or did they? It cannot be established now, but there is little evidence that there was recourse to the law for a woman who did object, but the husband of a woman who was raped could sue for damages (to his property?). One could sum up this millennium as a time of rape and incest.

As the Church grew stronger one of its first objectives was to make the idea of monogamous marriage its prime concern, and the Anglo Saxon Synod of 786 reinforced this when it decreed that the illegitimate son was not eligible to inherit. Following this it was able to bring in stricter and stricter regulations with virginity being more and more seen as the ideal situation. This being the case, it was a very blessed state for a wife to refuse her husband, which obviously led to a number of men finding solace outside the home. Sex within marriage was severely curtailed. It was illegal on sundays, wednesdays and fridays, and for 40 days before Easter, 40 days after Christmas, 40 days after giving birth, three days before Communion and three days after Communion as well as at any time of penance. It is not hard to see that a recipe for personal unhappiness, repression and neurosis was being brewed.

The next step for the Church was to ban all forms of sexual expression except intercourse within marriage for the reason of procreation. Fornication at this time was deemed to be a greater sin than murder. One act of fornication was held by the venerable Bede to require a penance for a year, whilst Dunstan's penalty for it was ten years of lamentation, fasting and abstention from meat. Fornication did not just include the sexual act. It encompassed kissing, nocturnal emissions, and even thinking about sex, but the worst thing of all according to Aquinas, was the practice of masturbation which was the greatest sin of all. (This was based on the sins of Onan, erroneously as it happens for his sin was actually coitus interruptus). Obviously this gave rise to a great number of taboos, not least of which were parental strictures in the case of infantile masturbation and one cannot help wondering how much repression in adults was directly related to this and in what way was it manifest. It is not difficult to see what the result was in one part of the population, the nuns and monks. The literature of the time is filled with accounts of nuns being visited by demons and incubi, and monks by succubi. The interesting thing about these manifestations is their similarity to the sexual act, i.e. the convulsions and arched bodies of the nuns (arc-en-circle). In Freudian terms it would be called an hysterical manifestation of the sexual act itself. Cynics would wonder how such virginal creatures would know how the sexual act was performed without prior knowledge. There were also accounts of erotomania focused on Jesus Himself, such as Margaretha of Ypern (1216-37) who believed herself to be engaged to Jesus (Rattray Taylor, 1953). The men tended to go in for self-flagellation and were particularly fond of hair shirts and some, such as Ammonius, took it further and regularly burned themselves with hot irons. The women tended to be masochistic in a different way. They seemed to go in for eating or drinking unpleasant things such as bitter herbs and ashes or dirty water.

The depressing thing about all this is the way the Church extolled these practices and in fact canonised some of the practitioners such as St Catherine, St Rose des Flores, St Dominic and St John of the Cross. The middle ages were a time of excess sexual regulation and this was particularly the case towards the sexuality of women. In past times women had been treated as property but now there was a move towards seeing her as the source of all sexual evil. Her body was likened to a cesspit and she was stigmatized as an agent of Satan and so began the unhealthy obsession with the minutiae of people's sexual lives that would ultimately culminate in the witch hunts. This period was predominately one of a patriarchal society, authoritarian, rule bound and restrictive where the tendency was for males to model themselves on their fathers and masculine traits were extolled.

Meanwhile another model was coming into its own which originated in the warm and sunny climate of the Languedoc of France. This was the age of the troubadours, or of courtly love, and it came to England under the influence of Eleanor of Aquitaine. The troubadours, instead of taking patriarchy as their role model, embraced the concept of matriarchy. They had the Virgin Mary as their patron and in fact instituted the feast of The Immaculate Conception. They conceived the idea of purity in love and sang songs to their mistresses who very often were married and whose husbands were the patrons of the troubadours. The women were seen as being more powerful and superior to the troubadour and his songs were filled with longing just to touch her, or even just her clothes. Rather than physical love, it was more a meeting of hearts and minds. The love that the troubadour focused on the lady of his choice was always pure, but that did not necessarily mean that he did not have a physical relationship with other women. Some writers have suggested that they were passive homosexuals and identified with women because of it. Whatever the truth of the matter the effect was to civilize attitudes towards women and bring in the concepts of honour and chivalry. The cult of the Virgin Mary followed on from this and towards the end of the 11th century an Ave (Rattray Taylor, 1953) was added to the Lord's Prayer. However, the strange thing was that whilst worshipping a Virgin could have deepened the sexual repression, the reverse became the case and the Virgin became rather like an older Earth Mother Goddess. She became a restorer of fertility and an aid to women in childbirth (another Juno Lucina?).

However, this was not enough to save women from another onslaught. No physical system could keep the people in order, terror was needed. Heaven was too insipid a concept, so Hell was made awful and there was an ever-increasing emphasis on damnation, and women were stigmatized as the agents of Satan. This began with the Papal Bull of Innocent VIII the 'Summa Desiderates Affectibus' of 1484. This was followed by the treatise of two Dominicans Sprenger and Kramer the `Malleus Maleficarum' of 1486 and so started the witchcraft mania or femicide that spread through Europe like wildfire. It was based upon the `fact' that `devils, incubi and succubi' ...`hinder men from performing the sexual act' (Thomas, 1971). Gradually these incubi and succubi were reduced to one gender - the female - and again the reason was one of sexuality. Women were accused of flying through the air (flying in dreams is always associated with sex) and of making men impotent. These women were always accused of taking part in some sexual practice with the Devil particularly that of the `obscene kiss'. It is interesting to note that the midwives of this time, who were lucky enough not to be accused, did not have a remedy for pain relief although they had a repertoire of charms and prayers and were knowledgeable about herbs. Was this because the most effective remedies, e.g. belladonna and atropine and the like were hallucinogens and caused visions and feelings of flying? The Malleus Maleficarum urged that midwives take an oath to eliminate any possibility of their resort to witchcraft. Midwives had always been 'the occasion of much superstition and dishonour of God' according to Bishop Latimer (Forbes, 1966) and so it is hardly surprising that those who survived steered clear from any suggestion of witchcraft. In fact the oath they took until the second half of the 18th century contained a promise to refrain from the use of sorcery and enchantment during the period of labour.

The century before the Papal Bull saw the start of the Renaissance and with it a disrespect for authority and a greater slide towards a matriarchy and away from the rule-bound authoritarianism of the Middle Ages. It brought with it a freer attitude to sex, social reforms and uninhibited attitude to learning. Women were unconstrained in their choice of clothes and generally the styles were gayer and more overtly sexual. These influences only started to affect England in Tudor times and strangely enough so did the Reformation which led to two contrary movements developing at the same time. In some ways they acted as a balance for one another. Sexual matters were less restricted than they had been but there was not a great movement towards licentiousness. Also Henry VIII had broken with Rome and had united the civil and ecclesiastical authorities. He also took sexual offences outside the jurisdiction of the Church e.g. sodomy now became a felony. Women also came into their own, sexually, as is shown in the writings of Shakespeare. Women were starting to take the lead in matters of sex and the dress of both sexes left one in no doubt as to their gender. This continued with the House of Stuart. Clothes for both sexes became more lavish with silks and lace and long coats. The court of James I was particularly permissive and it is said that this was in part due to his homosexuality. There was during this time a revival of the old fertility games, such as the May day festivities and the Easter fertility entertainments.

This pattern seesawed for the next few hundred years with the ascendancy of Puritanism and then the Restoration. The first caused a repression which attempted to restrict pleasure of all types and was particularly focused on immorality. In Freudian terms they were trying to operate always in the super ego mode and attempted to keep it in control by decrying drink and the theatre, or anything else which might bring feelings to the fore. In some respects, rather than repressing sex it was sublimated into the work ethic and consequently they did make many economic advances. When the Restoration was complete with Charles II on the throne, a new era of pleasure came in, but it was also characterized by unscrupulousness and violence. Brawls and fights seemed to go hand in hand with sexuality. Defloration became almost a national sport. It seemed that there was still the underlying resentment to women, as much of the literature shows in its obsession with the victims struggles and cries. It was also a time of prostitution on a large scale with virgins being extremely highly prized (and priced). It was, all in all, an age of failure to sublimate the sexual libido and one where there was an excessive need for sexual stimulation. Women were of contradictory status. Although they enjoyed much personal freedom and were beginning to make names for themselves as writers, poets and thinkers they were still faced with the old underlying threats. It was an age of perversion and prostitution and cavalier behaviour towards women.

It was followed by a swing back to patriarchy and the introduction of Romanticism and a swing back to a Romanticized era. This was the age of the twin soul theory and led up to the Victorian age. The theory was based on the Greek ideas of the function of women - for sex, for company and for bearing children. However unlike the Greeks who had three types of women to fulfil these functions - the slaves, the hetaerae and the wives - the Romantic ideal was to have all three encompassed by one woman. To some extent this idea is still around, for it is not unusual for men to want a wife who is a cook in the kitchen, a partner in the business and a whore in bed. This was the era of the great Romantic poets and Shelley and Byron particularly spring to mind. This seemed to be an age which was in reaction to patriarchy and father identification. It was the age of freer sexual morality and a higher status for women, but it gradually declined as the Victorian age took hold.

This was an age of double standards. There was an outer shell of moral rectitude, prudery and family values, whilst within there was a frightening amount of exploitation, suffering and deception. It was the age of the sexless woman and the child prostitute, the era of authoritarianism and of Darwin. The Victorians considered themselves civilized and above the savages whom they made it their business to enlighten, but they had one big problem, that of male sexuality. It was thought to bind men to an animal level and 'became the focus of a more generalized fear of disorder and of a continuing battle to tame natural forces' (Douglas, 1975). Middle- and upper-class men fought a constant battle with themselves to maintain their positions of power within society and within their homes and so were constantly on guard. They feared pollution and disorder from below and sexuality from within. So it was necessary for them to form a twin image of women who must be either madonnas or whores i.e. a female was either a lady, who was good and sexless, or she was a woman, who was none of these. This fitted into the culture and religion of the time very neatly. This was the age of the nature/culture debate and as women were seen as nearer to nature they were obviously subordinate and dangerous. Women's carnality was also a keystone of Christian theology. This splitting into opposite stereotypes caused great psychological problems because love was split into the sacred and the profane. The sexual act 'was seen as something degrading which defiles and pollutes not only the body' (Freud, 1977). So men did not want to defile their wives or be defiled by them, which left them with quite a problem as the other notable value of the Victorian era was that of family. So the answer to the dilemma was to desexualize the wife, who now was doing her duty against unpleasant odds and to carnalize the subordinate working-class women. They being nearer to nature were thought to be without morals and to be both fair game and willing whatever their age. Another feature of this preoccupation and of the double standards was the preoccupation with symbols and euphemisms (a whole language of `gloves' arose from this) as well as verbal representations, e.g. childbirth was now referred to as accouchement. Another sad thing for women was the lack of interest and indeed firm opposition to pain relief in childbirth. Due to the Church's position regarding the role of women, the taking of chloroform by Queen Victoria did not pass lightly.

The past 90 years have seen a movement towards sexual reform for women. It probably began albeit unwittingly with Havelock Ellis (1959). He was amongst the first to consider sexuality as a concept and although he did have a romanticized view of it and was in total agreement with the current thinking that sexuality was male, he did recognize (obliquely) the importance of the clitoris. Generally, if female sexuality was considered at all it was the vagina that was mythologized (or eulogized) in defence of the penis as the organ of sex. The 20th century has seen the beginnings of the movement to reconstruct the female as a sexual being. Frigidity and fertility control were the areas fought over in the early part of the century for they underpinned other more political debates, those of virginity, extramarital sex and the rights of women over their own bodies. In short they were preoccupied with sexual and political repression of women.

Women who were not satisfied within the sexual relationship were 'frigid'. Dickinson and Beam (1932) found pain and maladjustment in a significant number of women. The responsibility was always the woman's, although it does take two to make love as well as to tango. Hirschfield (1953) as recently as 1953 warned of the devastating effects on men of women's frigidity. Failure to reach orgasm as well as the avoidance of pregnancy preoccupied the women who attended Marie Stopes and Janet Chance's marriage advisory clinics (Stopes and Chance, 1952). A sexual revolution for women started quietly with writers such as Simone De Beauvoir (1953) who pointed out the flaws in the sexual reformer's arguments that women were at the heart of all heterosexual problems. She pointed out the importance of the clitoris and welcomed sexual activity for pleasure alone i.e. unrelated to pregnancy, unfettered by worries about pregnancy and unchained from monogamy.

13

The years that followed saw the publication of the Kinsey report in 1953 followed by the growth of the Women's Liberation Movement. Kinsey's report had major implications for women's sexuality because not only did it challenge the myth of the vagina as the seat of female orgasm, it rejected the Freudian notion of the clitoris as an immature organ. This was followed by the permissive sixties and the writers of the era such as Masters and Johnson (1966) and Germaine Greer (1969) affirming woman as a sexual being in her own right. This was linked in to the politics of the day and in England had an influence on the struggle to gain more autonomy and equal rights for women. Even so there was still a relentless use of women's bodies by the marketing and sex industries, to sell anything from soap powder and cars, to the vicarious relief of the solitary. In obstetrics those fundamental aspects of female sexuality, pregnancy, labour and childbirth were seen as the domain of the patriarchs and the seventies saw a massive rise in the technology and medicalization of the birthing process. The 1980s and '90s have seen the rise of the sexually transmitted disease AIDS (auto immune deficiency syndrome), which has given rise to a new wave of Puritanical preaching. Now gay men and promiscuous heterosexuals are at the receiving end of phobia. It is too soon to tell whether it will lead to a new era of restriction and virginity cults. If one was to refer to past centuries it would seem unlikely because the Church does not have the power it once had and the threat of hellfire and damnation is not a modern enough concept. However fear of women and their sexuality is such an ingrained part of the national psyche that it is not impossible for women to lose ground once more in the move towards sexual equality and of course gay men can be accused of hedonism, always a threat to the super ego.

CHAPTER TWO

The Making of Man and Woman

So God created man in His own image, in the image of God He created him;
male and female He created them.
Genesis Ch.1, v.27

Are men and women the products of biological givens, or are they the products of a cultural construction? This question may seem strange to anyone to anyone who thinks in terms of absolutes. However if one thinks of gender as the ascribed position in society that a person bearing certain anatomical features are placed then it seems more relevant. 'A gender system is a symbolic or meaning system that consists of two complementary yet exclusive categories into which all human beings are placed' (Cucchiari, cited in Ortner and Whitehead, 1981) and the genitals are the sole criteria for assigning a person to a category at birth. This is very evident in the labour room, usually the first declaration from the midwife, the father or the mother herself is 'it's a girl' or 'it's a boy' and is followed by the question, 'Is she [or he] alright'. From that moment the pathway of the individual's life is set. She or he is either feminine or masculine. The congratulatory cards, the baskets of flowers and the gifts of clothes are sent in shades of pink for a girl or blue for a boy, and so it goes on for the rest of life. This categorization only happens once in an individual's life and so the person, particularly if a midwife or doctor, must be absolutely confident that they have got it right. In the case of ambiguous genitalia the decision to assign the infant to a category is usually deferred until further biological tests are done and although this can be harrowing it is not as problematic as when a mistake is made. Even if the mistake is rectified after a very short time there will be problems for the family and the infant in particular. It will always have a history (however short) of blurred gender identity with greater or lesser effects.

At one time girls were given dolls and ironing boards to play with and boys were given miniature tool kits and guns. Even in the progressive

'90s when there is a move to give gender neutral toys and to send little girls signals that they can have such things as a car, and that boys can cook and do not (or should not) necessarily have to be fighters, the gender messages are still there albeit in a more subtle way. It is well-documented by child psychologists that mothers treat little boys differently from girls (Lewis, 1975). Boys tend to be praised for different behavioural characteristics, such as boisterousness, which is tolerated and encouraged in boys more than girls.

Gender is the classification of rules, meanings and categories that society places men and women into and so is as diverse as the cultures of the world. Universally speaking there are only two genders recognized (except perhaps for the Navajo who recognize a third, 'the nadle', or intersex who may or may not be a hermaphrodite). This Universal dichotomy only means that there are two classifications within that society not that societies are alike or even at times similar. The biological anatomical difference is not the only criterion for the definition of gender. Additional features are constructed by different cultures such as temperament, fate, ability and cosmology. This can be illustrated by the significance of the dreaming of a pregnant Mohave Indian, if she dreams of the bow strap it will be a boy and if a burden strap it will be a girl. Having other criteria means that although there are only two genders, there can be mixing or seeping which leads to a muddled gender status. For example in New Guinea young boys are 'deficient' in gender, and so homosexuality may be appropriate in certain circumstances (Ortner and Whitehead, 1981) whereas in Western Society homosexuality is generally seen as gender crossing rather than a true difference in gender. There are two key features to the gender model, sex and reproduction and from these is built up a complex framework involving the classification, assignment, identity, role and stereotypes of gender.

Before going into detail about the gender issues it may be useful to say something about the biological basis of gender, i.e. sex and its determinants.

Every cell in the human body is a diploid cell containing 46 chromosomes. These chromosomes carry the genetic message of the individual. There are 44 autosomes in 22 homologous pairs which carry information from both parents. One chromosome in every pair is derived from the mother and one from the father. Each chromosome has genes arranged linearly along its length and the genes are responsible for a characteristic. If a gene is identical in one chromosome to its opposite on the other chromosome, the person is said to be homozygous for that characteristic, but if they are not the same, the person is heterozygous for that characteristic. In some cases one gene's characteristic masks the other's and is said to be dominant and the masked gene is recessive. The actual genetic makeup of a person is called their genotype and how they are expressed is their phenotype. For example, a brown-eyed person may be genotype heterozygous, i.e. he or she carries both the gene for blue eyes and for brown, but because the gene for brown eyes is dominant his or her phenotype is for brown eyes. He or she will be indistinguishable from a person who is both phenotype and homozygous genotype for brown eyes.

In addition to the 44 autosomes, each individual carries a pair of chromosomes which differ from the autosomes in that it is only in the female that they are homologous XX, in the male they are heterologous XY. These are the 'sex' chromosomes and determine what kind of reproductive cell the mature individual will carry. Although the genetic sex of an individual is determined at the time of conception, it is only at about the eighth week that it becomes apparent. This is when the medulla of the gonads in the abdominal cavity start to develop into the testes in the male due to the influence of the Y chromosome and its production of the androgen hormones. When there are two X chromosomes the medulla will develop into ovaries which by the 12th week of gestation will contain all the ova that will ever be produced by that individual. There are two sets of ducts in the embryo, they are the Mullerian and the Wolffian ducts. After the testes have formed at about eight weeks they produce a substance (possibly an androgen) which inhibits the development of the Mullerian ducts and causes their eventual atrophy. At about three months gestation the androgens cause the Wolffian ducts to develop and form the seminal vesicles, the ejaculatory ducts and the vas deferens. Without the influence of the androgens the Mullerian ducts continue to develop and become the fallopian tubes, the uterus and the vagina, whilst the Wolffian ducts atrophy. Androgens also affect the external genitalia causing the penis to form and the labia to fuse forming the scrotum. This can happen when for some reason, e.g. in the salt losing adreno genital syndrome high levels of androgens are formed by a female fetus and the baby at birth is of indeterminate sex due to virilization of the female external genitalia, a case of intersex or hermaphroditism. In intrauterine life the development of the internal and external genitalia is complete by the 16th week in the male and by the 20th week in the female. There is a low and steady secretion of androgens and oestrogens throughout childhood until about the age of 11 or 12 when puberty starts.

At puberty due to a combination of imperfectly understood factors such as critical body weight, there begins an increase in the sex hormones. In the female the hypothalamus produces a substance, gonadotrophin releasing hormone, which acts on the anterior pituitary gland, causing it to produce follicle stimulating hormone which induces follicle development within the ovary. Each month one ovum outstrips the others in its development and is eventually released into the fallopian tube to journey towards the spermatozoa and fertilization. Developing ova produce oestrogen, which in turn inhibits the production of follicle stimulating hormone and facilitates the release of luteinizing hormone from the anterior pituitary gland. This in its turn causes the production of progesterone from the corpus luteum, i.e. the cells surrounding the maturing ovum. In addition to instigating this menstrual cycle, the hormones cause the development of the breasts, the uterus and the vagina, deposition of fat around the hips and buttocks, and the production of pubic and axillary hair. In the male the testes produce greater amounts of androgens causing the development of bone and muscle, enlargement of the larynx (the voice deepens and 'breaks'), enlargement of the penis and testicles, production of seminal fluid and spermatozoa and the growth of facial, body, pubic and axillary hair.

Although there are two biological sexes there can be anomalies of combinations of sex chromosomes. These anomalies all have one factor in common they contain an X chromosome which seems necessary for life. They develop from an abnormality in the gamete such as XO (Turner's syndrome) where there is only one sex chromosome, the X. This individual develops into a normal female but at puberty fails to menstruate or significantly develop secondary sex characteristics. She is usually normal in every other way. With XXY (Klinefelter's syndrome), the person has underdeveloped male genitalia, is sterile and is usually mentally retarded. With XYY the person is a normal biological male in every way. None of the anomalies have been found to cause other than 'normal' gender identities, i.e. they have not been associated with transsexualism. (Money, Hampson and Hampson, 1955). XXX females are not 'more' feminine and XO females 'less' feminine than 'ordinary' XX females nor are XYY males 'more' manly than XY males. In everyday life gender is usually ascribed on physical attributes rather than on chromosomes except in one instance, that of the Olympic games. Originally women were barred from the games in Ancient Greece and a simple gender test was instituted - the athletes competed naked. Now there is a much more sophisticated process in place, the competitor has to pass a chromosome test. Unfortunately the cells are examined for Barr bodies and the number of Barr bodies in a cell is one less than the number of X chromosomes. This means that a female with the genetic makeup XO who is most definitely not a male will have no Barr bodies just as a man with XY chromosomes will not. The original reason for instituting the tests was to prevent a man from posing as a female because males are 'naturally' stronger than females. However with the increasing number of women who workout in the gym to develop very strong physiques it can now be shown that strength is not sex-linked. There is also another factor to be considered in the testing and ascribing of gender to chromosome makeup, that of mosaic patterns i.e. some individuals have some cells with XO and others with XY and so on, which could make their gender even more of a subjective decision.

If gender is classified through the recognition of the external genitalia and further reinforced by other factors such as the horoscope or fate then one is still left with the question of identity. Is the identity of the individual as a man or a woman a biological given or is it a construction? Behavioural variations begin to manifest themselves towards the end of the first year of life. It has been suggested (Garai and Scheinfeld, 1968) that there are some differences which manifest themselves very early and point to a biological distinction, but this has been discredited due to unreliable and inconsistent evidence from study to study (Archer and Lloyd, 1987). Even if behavioural differences were found very early on in baby boys and girls, it would not necessarily follow that they were a result of biological sex differences (*op. cit.*). The classic study by Moss (1970) showed that mother's interacted longer with their baby boys at birth than with their baby girls but progressively less at three months, although the differential was still there. It was observed that the baby boys were 'crankier' (i.e. more bad-tempered) at birth than the girls and the explanation was put forward that boys may have behavioural difficulties due to their greater vulnerability at birth and the greater risk of complications. This was not the whole story because it was noted that where babies were in similar states of arousal the mothers seemed to stimulate the boys more, but responded to the girls by imitation and feedback. This may help to explain the verbal superiority of the female infant. White and Wollett in a further study in 1981 also found that adults differentiate between boys and girls from birth onwards but again this does not prove a biological determinant.

It can be proved in laboratory studies with rodents that testosterone secreted in early fetal life affects behaviour in extrauterine life, but obviously this cannot be prospectively reproduced in the human. However Money and Erhardt (1972) pioneered research in this area and follow-up studies by Baker in 1980 and Erhardt, Ince and Mayer-Bahlberg in 1981 showed that females prenatally exposed to androgens were likely to exhibit more 'tomboyish' behaviour than girls who had not. These studies were not met with unanimous agreement for it was pointed out (Quadagno, Briscoe and Quadagno, 1977) that some of the girls in the studies received late correction for genital abnormalities and this brings us to the nature/nurture (or nature/culture) debate.

If there are no biological determinants then gender and by extension sexuality must be an instituted process. John Money (1965) goes further and maintains that men and women come into the world as bisexual beings and restrictions on sexuality are largely due to cultural partitions. Although each culture does it differently it is usually within the gender system. All the prohibitions are about normative statements, i.e. what is right about men and women - gender statements. If human sexuality is plastic then heterosexuality is a restriction, or as Ortner and Whitehead (1981) would have it, an incest taboo. It may be that the earliest form of institutional normalization is within the family but it is much wider and well within the public domain. It is here that the edges are blurred between nurture and culture.

Culture is the wealth of rules, meanings and symbols that are handed down in society in order to make sense of and survive in the world. Nurture is far more personal and within the family in that it is more often associated with the protection, care and upbringing of the children. In many ways the nurturing influence is that of handing down the culture. What is often seen and has been discussed at length by Ortner (1973) is that men are viewed in most cultures as nearer to culture and women nearer to nature. Some cultures, such as those found in Meditteranean countries, have highly elaborated ideas of gender and sexuality and these views organize and define other spheres of life. In some cultures although they have definite gender systems they are not necessarily symmetrical. For example, there may be definite patterns of life for men but not for women, such as rites of passage.

There are many cultures which have highly complex rituals for boys to become men but little for girls on becoming women. This may be due to the biological evidence of a girl's maturity - menstruation - or it may really be reflecting the lack of importance of women in public life. Ardener (1978) says that women are invisible and this invisibility is, refracted through and embedded in many different social spaces: in seating arrangements, economic patterns, status, value and symbolic systems, and so forth and the phenomenon of men speaking for women causes no comment.

If one sees the domestic domain or the family as the biological entity, as Levi-Strauss (1969) did, and the wider network of social interactions as 'culture' then it becomes easier to see why women are more closely linked with nature and men with culture. The problem is that they are seen as diametrically opposed and just as nature has to be subdued in order that man can prosper so women in this metaphor must be subdued also. According to Ortner (1974) all women in all societies are valued at a lower level than men and she came to the conclusion that the reason for this is their reproductive capacity. It brings them nearer to nature because they are primarily associated with the rearing of children who are pre-social or not yet culturally complete. As man must transcend and control nature in order to survive, women being symbolically at one with nature must be treated the same. (In reality women are no nearer or further from nature than men.) This leads to many and various restrictions on women's sexuality and reproductive capacity, but also, and perhaps more damaging for women, it has lead to the conceptualization of men and women as a set of oppositions. So if men are 'up', women are 'down', and if men are 'strong', women are 'weak', and so it goes on. The most overwhelming opposition is that if men are 'public' women are 'private' and so men are involved in the wider sphere of society and the greater good whilst women are involved with the family and with the particularistic. This can be seen in the different attitudes in the literature to war; men are portrayed as going out to fight for Queen and Country, whilst women stay at home and weep and pray for their sons. The other damaging aspect of the nature/culture debate for women is the concept of pollution. Blood is very frightening as its presence is often a harbinger of death and a reminder of man's mortality and so woman with her monthly flow and the blood of childbirth poses yet another threat. So in many cultures woman is surrounded by many behavioural taboos and restrictions and very often isolated from the main living areas when menstruating. This polluting effect gives women power, which in itself cause a dilemma because how can a powerless, controlled person have power. The answer is simple. It has to be the wrong sort of power which again needs to be controlled. As Mary Douglas (1992) points out, 'a polluting person is always in the wrong'. The polluting person is not the same as a witch or sorcerer who are malicious, for pollution can be set off inadvertently. This being so it can be seen why women are so dangerous, for after all they prepare the food, and have to be enclosed until they have been ritually purified (for example in the Jewish Mikvah).

Men tend to be defined by their occupation such as warrior, hunter, engineer, bus driver, whereas women are most often described in relationship terms as mother, sister or wife. In many societies women are also defined by the amount of control that there is over their sexuality, the virgin princess will be the most controlled woman in a patrilineal society where it is important for men to know who their children are. Aspects of kinship and marriage most definitely enter into any thinking about gender and gender roles. Gender roles are the sets of prescriptions and proscriptions about behaviour that are laid down for the person in a specific social context. These are so rigidly adhered to that they actually form a set of expectations about what is appropriate behaviour. In fact the Collins English dictionary 1986 edition so closely links the definition of woman with her role that it uses the example of 'babies bring out the woman in her' to explain what a woman is.

Expectations about gender behaviour tend to fall, unsurprisingly, into two opposite camps. These behaviours are evaluated as good, bad, desirable or undesirable. For example, men are seen to be ambitious, forceful, good at science and do not cry. They go to work to feed their families so their work is valued and highly paid. Women in contrast are carers, they are gentle, kind and sentimental and their fulfilment is found within the home, working to keep the family comfortable, so that any work they do outside the home is of secondary importance and can be paid at a lower rate than 'men's' work. Obviously this is written with the understanding that these roles are stereotypes and probably do not exist in such concentrated measure for everyone all the time. However, one cannot dismiss stereotypes as being unreal, because they do fit in with the mass idea of a reality somewhere (even if it is not for oneself). These ideas in actual fact reflect the invisibility of women rather than their contribution to the labour market, for a cursory examination of any society will show quite clearly that women's work is indispensable (even in hunter gatherer societies it is more likely that the gatherers will provide a constant supply of food, as well as preparing it, looking after the children and gathering fuel.)

As expectations of behaviour are so entrenched in society there are strict sanctions against people who do not conform. Men do not wear dresses in the street except in certain areas of the town where it is safe to do so. Women do not make love to their women partners in public places. Less extremely, women do not display 'male'-type behaviour such as aggression and naked ambition without having to pay a price for it, and men who prefer to stay at home and bring up the children whilst their wives work are likewise viewed with suspicion. In the 1990s things are changing and there is blurring of the edges in the gender dichotomy, but it is the sanctions that are being eroded away rather than an abandonment of the fundamental stereotypes. (This is very evident in the Equal Opportunities Legislation.) Having said that, there is an increasing tendency to challenge the prevailing assumptions and the dichotomous nature of gender roles which has led to the 'New Man' of the '80s and '90s. How new the 'New Man' really is remains a matter for conjecture, because one suspects that even within the most modern and liberal of domestic set-ups there are patterns of behaviour which are still gender biased, for example, control of the television remote control is often a male-dominated behaviour.

Although there is not a strict categorization of interests, hobbies and activities into opposing gender categories there are some that are more male than female and vice versa. For example, women play tennis and watch rugby, they swim and go fell-walking, and men write poetry and go horse riding. Except for a few activities such as boxing and knitting the activities in themselves are gender neutral, but there is a tendency to group like with like and categorize an individual from the activities that he or she enjoys. For example, a feminine (or effeminate) person stereotypically likes to knit and sew, watch television and wear makeup, whilst the masculine (or butch) person will play football, go mountaineering and likes to tinker with cars. The problem here lies in the internal world of the person. As society's attitudes to gender differences are so rigid, there may be difficulties for people who enjoy the 'wrong' interests. Just because they have the biological signs of one sex they have been ascribed a set of behavioural assumptions that they are forced to live with for the rest of their lives. It may be that it is not a problem for most people, but for some it can be a heavy burden. At the extreme end there may be people who are so uncomfortable with their ascribed gender that they will cross dress, or they may go even further and have surgery in an effort to cross the boundary (see Chapter 11); but most will continue in their ascribed gender and may fulfil the social obligations, such as having children, but still remain, if not an oddity, somewhat different.

If society for the most part makes such a good job of sorting people out into two categories perhaps it will be useful to look at how it is done. Apart from the psychoanalytical view, which will be looked at in Chapter 3, there are two main theories, that of social development and that of cognitive development.

The social development theory is based on the principle of identification. Studies of parent-child interaction (Kessler and McKenna, 1987) show that children identify with their parents and other significant adults. Identification is defined as the imitation and incorporation of complex values and behaviours without specific external pressure to do this. There are other factors involved, such as direct teaching and pressure by individuals and institutions to act in a certain way. There is a pattern of reward, non-reward and punishment that is used. So the child learns because he or she sees the parent as a powerful and effective force in their lives. The child learns the word 'boy' or 'girl' in association with appropriate behaviour. For example, the boy is told he is a brave boy for not crying when he falls down or conversely is told not to be a crybaby girl. The girl is told she is a pretty little girl and told not to get dirty. The assumption is that children want rewards and as they are rewarded for gender-appropriate behaviours they will continue in them. Having said that, a girl may not wear frilly, pretty-pretty clothes when she grows up, but she will know she is a girl. That will remain unchallenged. The social development theory does not concern itself too much with ideas in that the idea of gender itself remains unexamined. It takes for granted that there are two genders based on objective criteria. It is not concerned about the acquisition of gender-type behaviour through cognitive processes but is mainly reliant on the reinforcement aspects.

A contrast to this is the cognitive theory which has as its base the work of Kohlberg and Ullian (1974) and Piaget (1952). Briefly this theory asserts that gender is a physical category based on anatomy and that until children have the concept of conservation as described by Piaget, they do not have permanent gender identities. Until they are about three years old children cannot label themselves accurately. According to Kohlberg, when they are about three years old they may be able to do so, but they will not know that gender is permanent or that everyone has a gender and that it is based on physical characteristics. They develop permanent gender identities at about six years old and start to identify with the parent of the same sex. Not only does a six-year-old girl know she is a girl, she also likes being that way. She identifies with her mother and prefers female activities and dress. Likewise the boy identifies with his father. As being masculine is seen by both sexes as powerful, girls identify with their fathers as well to some extent. This theory emphasizes the child's active role in structuring the world according to his or her level of cognitive development. It is based on the work of Piaget in that it states that the reality of a child is very different from that an adult. Piaget said that the child sees the world in discrete stages until he becomes an adult and sees it 'accurately'. Accuracy is a very debatable word and it is probably more true to say that the child develops until it shares the same rules for constructing the world as adults do. The work of both Kohlberg and Piaget have been criticised in other contexts but for the work on gender there are three main criticisms. The first is that a child may be able to label a person as male and or female, but may not really know the difference. Secondly, it is not necessary for a child to be cognitively aware of gender differences to be socialized into the role. Thirdly, the theory of cognitive development will not stand alone without the concept of reinforcement.

In the preceding discussion of gender and its construction, one aspect of gender was briefly alluded to and passed over. This was the female's property of reproduction, i.e. motherhood. Motherhood is itself a social construction and differs from society to society. In the West, and in Britain particularly, it has undergone several major changes in the past 90 years or so. Just as childhood is a recent phenomenon and in fact does not exist apart from a biological reality in other parts of the modern world, so the concept of exclusive mothering is new. There is an idea in modern Western society that a mother is a woman who is filled with maternal instinct and overwhelming love for her child from the moment of birth. She then proceeds to stay, isolated at home with her child, providing her or him with constant care and moral and social guidance. This is not true for the vast majority of women now and never has been. Before the Factory Acts in England, working class women and children were very necessary to the economy as workers, and upper and middle class women employed surrogate mothers in one form or another. One of these, the nanny, still exists in parts of English society today. The concept alters to fit the circumstances. For example in the last World War children were evacuated to the country to live with complete strangers whilst their mothers were exhorted to work in the munitions factories or on the land as part of the war effort. In addition there were day nurseries in every locality. However, in the post-war years in an effort to restore the status quo and return men to jobs, the spectre of the 'latch-key kid' was foisted upon women. Dire consequences were forecast for children whose mothers went out to work. This ideology did not take into account the vast numbers of stable, law abiding children brought up by working war widows or by single professional women. There is another twist to the tale in the present-day context. Now it is not enough for the mother to stay at home and look after the child exclusively, another rider has been added. If the mother is single and living on State benefits, she must be encouraged to return to work, or better still marry and fulfil the new dream of a return to the 'traditional' nuclear family.

Stanworth (1988) would argue that the construction of motherhood is changing yet again due to the rise of the reproductive technologies. On the one hand, there is a powerful ideology that states that motherhood is the natural goal of all women and to deny one's maternal instinct is selfish, peculiar or disturbed. This is so entrenched in the medical profession's thinking as to be presented as a fact, for example, 'It is a fact that there is a biological drive to reproduce. Women who deny this drive, or in whom it is frustrated, show disturbance in other ways' (Steptoe, in Stanworth, 1987). It is also very true for a great number of women who on an individual level do want to be mothers. This being so they are willing to undergo any amount of treatment, medication or surgery to achieve this state. Motherhood alone is not sufficient, for if it was, adoption would resolve the matter. One train of feminist thinking (the structuralist) (Hubbard, 1985) maintains that there is no biological desire to reproduce, but that it is a social construction which has been used to keep women in a domestic role. According to Beauvoir (1953) the fundamental fact that from the beginning of history doomed women to domestic work and 'prevented her from taking part in the shaping of the world was her enslavement to the generative function'. This ideology gives rise to two problems for feminist thinkers. The first is that the technologies can and should give autonomy to women. They should now become mistresses of their own fertility, i.e. they should now be able to commandeer the resources of the technologies to prevent conception or have an abortion if they so wish. They should also be able to achieve motherhood on their own terms, without male partners for instance. As they patently are not in control of this situation it is seen as a reduction in autonomy and enslavement by a hegemonistic medical profession which represents male domination of women. The other problem is that of indoctrination into the ideology which causes suffering for infertile women. As Corea (1992) says of those that repeatedly operate and experiment on women, 'they are not asking how much of women's suffering has been socially constructed and inflicted and is therefore not inevitable'. Medical treatment only exacerbates the suffering and is generally lengthy, painful and ineffective and also by offering increasingly extreme technologies it makes the option to choose non-motherhood more difficult. Poff (1987) says that in order to have a meaningful alternative both women and men need to stop believing that childbearing is essential to the definition and nature of being a woman.

CHAPTER THREE

Sexuality, Theory or Praxis?

O that you would kiss me with the kisses of your mouth!
For your love is better than wine, your anointing oils are fragrant,
The Song of Solomon Ch.1, v.2

The primary theory of gender development, the psychoanalytical approach of Sigmund Freud, which was referred to in Chapter 2, not only bridges the gap between the work on gender development and the empiricists study of sexology, but has formed the basis for a wider understanding of sexuality. Freud was so prolific in his work and his writings that no account of sexuality would be complete without an examination of his thinking.

Freud, along with Havelock Ellis and Hirschfield, 'broke up the conspiracy of silence that had so largely stifled discussion in the nineteenth century, and at last awarded it with its rightful place in psychology and sociology' (Weeks, 1983). The difficulty, as was pointed out later by the feminist critics, was that the view was essentially male. Freud's attempts to understand the unconscious through the examination of his patient's dreams and fantasies led him to reach his radical view of sexuality which he published in 1905 in his `Three Essays on Sexuality' (Freud, 1986a). He set about studying the unconscious or primary process. It is interesting to note that the secondary process or conscious mind obeys the laws of logic, and critics of the feminist stance such as Mitchell (1974), point out that it is by applying the rules of logic that feminists find the theory wanting. It seems ironic that women who are normally accused of being illogical are also in the wrong when they take the logical approach (a case of heads you win, tails I lose?).

The baby is primarily a hedonistic creature which exists to satisfy its cravings, which are in the main for food and comfort. This, Freud terms the pleasure principle or the id. The id is the mass of primitive instincts and energies in the unconscious mind that is modified by the ego and super ego, but underlies all psychical activity. As he develops and begins to recognize the outer world a reality principle starts to arise, the ego. The ego is the self of the individual, the conscious state of mind, which is based on the perception of the environment from birth onwards. It is responsible for modifying the antisocial instincts of the id and is itself modified by the conscience or super ego which is an internal ideal of personal perfection, i.e. what one wants to be rather than what one is. It develops under the influence of superior powers, particularly those of the parents, and it sits in judgement on the ego leading to self observation, moral conscience and repression. The distance between the ego and the super ego varies greatly from person to person, at different stages in his or her life. Even after the ego and the super ego are well developed they do not replace the id. Desires, wants and feelings that are not acceptable to the world of reality do not go away, they are simply kept in the unconscious and repressed. The unconscious is made up of latent thought processes independent from the conscious mind and may even run counter to it (this has been shown by post-hypnotic suggestion). Active psychical forces or energy prevent unconscious thought from being summoned into the conscious.

Most of the unconscious is repressed and seeks expression in other ways, such as dreams, where thoughts from the day mingle with the unconsciousness. Three things happen in a dream, thoughts undergo transformation; they occupy the conscious mind when they should not and the unconscious pushes through to mingle with the thoughts. It was from dreams that Freud obtained much of his data, and it was from the concept of the id that he formulated his theory and explanation of human sexuality as developing from a polymorphous perverse infant sexuality to an adult heterosexual sexuality. He saw sexuality as an instinct and it may be useful to explain what in Freudian terms is an instinct. It is a stimulus to the mind which is not from an external source (e.g. light falling on the retina causes a reaction). The organism can withdraw or flee from this type of stimulus but it cannot flee from an instinct which is more akin to the feeling of thirst when the oesophagus has dried up. It is a constant driving force from which the organism cannot flee but must attempt to satisfy at all cost, and it is always active.

The sexual instinct was thought to be an impulse which attempts to bring the male and female genitalia into contact. It is easier to discuss the sexual instinct rather than sexuality, because even Sigmund himself got into a muddle when trying to define sexuality itself. In his Lecture XX after an initial attempt he neatly fudged the issue by concluding that, 'on the whole, indeed, we know pretty well what is meant by sexual' (Freud, 1933). He postulated that the sexual instinct starts just after birth and is not connected with the genitalia. It is a wider concept. Babies are polymorphous or bisexual, and gain sensual pleasure from many body areas including the mouth, the anus, the penis or the clitoris. The fundamental function of sexuality is to obtain pleasure from the zones of the body which Freud termed erotogenous zones, the first of which is the mouth. Although Freud (1986a) (p.99) confessed to not knowing what the stimuli were that produced the pleasurable feelings he did note that there had to be a rhythmic quality to them and that the original sensation had to be experienced physiologically to leave behind a residual need for it to continue. In infancy the child gains pleasure from its body and the process climaxes at the fifth year of life when there is a lull until puberty.

The infantile sexual process has three phases the oral, the anal and the phallic. The oral phase, the aim of which is to gain pleasure by the mouth, is undifferentiated in both sexes. It develops from the rooting and sucking instincts and the object is the breast (or autoerotically the child's own thumb). In the anal stage there is more control over the function and Freud talks about children who hold back their faeces as a means of both exhibiting aggression towards their 'nurse' and as a means of sexual gratification for themselves Freud, 1986b) . It is, in his mind, related to the development of sadism which is a fusion of pure libidinal and pure destructive impulses. The third phase of childhood is the phallic phase which starts at about the age of five years. Initially both sexes think about sex a great deal and assume the universal presence of the penis. In females excitation is from the clitoris which corresponds to the penis (Freud's phallocentric viewpoint).

Now, however, they proceed in different directions because one has 'it' and the other does not. The boy enters the Oedipal phase, which in 'Totem and Taboo' Freud (1913) suspects 'the sense of guilt of mankind as a whole, which is the ultimate source of religion and morality, was acquired in the beginning of history through the Oedipus complex'. (Oedipus in Greek mythology was the son of Laius and Jocasta, the king and queen of Thebes. Oedipus, not realizing who they were, killed his father and married his mother. They had four children together and on finding out the truth he put out his own eyes and his wife/mother Jocasta committed suicide.)

The boy now wants his mother all to himself, he falls in love with her and wants to marry her. He handles his genitals and fantasizes about her and becomes jealous of his father, who is now in the way. He shows his satisfaction when his father is absent, but has ambivalent feelings because he loves his father as well. His parent's reaction is to threaten him with castration and fearing this (which could be a reality, for he knows that girls have no penis, or it could be left over from prehistory when fathers would actually castrate their sons) he withdraws into the latency period. Following the stress due to the fear of castration the boy will give up masturbation but does not give up his fantasies. These early fantasies are modified and later play a part in the formation of the boy's character. In some way he identifies with his mother and a feminine aspect to his character is formed. In extreme cases it may leave him with an extreme dependence on his mother. He will repress much of this feeling but will become extremely submissive towards women in general. At puberty all these repressed feelings may re-emerge in an incoherent form and the young man will be torn by mutually conflicting impulses. This can be so deep that even in psychoanalysis it will be resisted.

Freud had difficulty with female sexuality and considered that girls feel the same as boys and have phallic dreams of penetration just as boys do. However their source of erotic feelings, the clitoris, he considered to be an inferior penis. Thus the sexuality of little girls is of a masculine character until they realize the inferiority of the penis, when it very often has a permanent effect on a girl's character and 'often after this initial disappointment she turns away from sexual life altogether' (Freud, 1905), and becomes frigid. She blames her mother for this `castration' and turns away from her, now identifying with her father. She envies the possession of the penis and tries to emulate the boy but when she does not gain the same satisfaction she gives up and gains a `normal' female sexuality. If she does not then she will remain envious of boys and become homosexual or she becomes annoyed with her mother and makes her father her love object. She wants to have her father's penis at her command and have a present from it (a baby). This Electra phase is resolved at puberty when the girl 'has accepted the passive nature of her sexuality and transferred the site of sexual pleasure from the clitoris to the vagina' (Chodorov, 1978). This is violently disputed by many of the feminist writers, for as Germaine Greer (1970) says,

The female genital organ, in keeping with the desexualization of her whole energy and the obliteration of her desire, became a mere hole, troops for the use of. Receptivity, which is no more passive an act than eating, became synonymous with passivity.

Likewise Simone De Beauvoir (1975) disagrees because,

> if women do envy men anything, it is most likely to be the almost exclusive hold on power that they have (which may be symbolized by the penis) rather than the penis itself.

By puberty the Oedipus or Electra phase is resolved in both sexes and two distinct patterns of sexuality have emerged. Boys develop an active type of sexuality and girls a passive one. Boys centre on penetration and impregnation of women, and girls centre on passivity and being penetrated with the ultimate aim of having a baby. The post-Oedipal child is understood in Freud's model to repress the earlier instincts and to fuse them into a mature structure. This repression can cause the instincts to be sublimated and channelled by the super ego into intellectual and artistic activities.

According to Freud this drive towards genital fixated heterosexuality sometimes goes awry and deviancy occurs. Some girls remain bisexual and do not want to become mothers. Such a woman may go one of two ways, she may become lesbian or neurotic. Boys may also become homosexual in the same way. A third possibility is that the person remains at a prephallic phase of sexual development and develops either an autoeroticism or an infantile fixation on objects. It has already been said this work was not and is not without its critics, the earliest being Horney (1924) who challenged the penis envy theory much as De Beauvoir was to do later by stating that it was the power of men not their appendage that women envied. These criticisms have been constant and reiterated by such different people as Melanie Klein (in Stockard and Johnson, 1979) and Kessler and McKenna (1978).

There are two further points to consider when evaluating Freud's theories and they are: first, that instincts as biological certainties cannot be proven and remain psychosocial concepts. Secondly, the primacy of the genitals may be culturally constructed and yet another example of the conquest of nature by socialization into the culture. This is a distinct possibility when one considers the extent that Freud used memories of past cultural events to generate data. If this is so then it also shows that human sexuality is not predetermined and neither genital heterosexual primacy nor bisexuality is inevitable.

In his 1905 work, 'Three Essays on the Theory of Sexuality' Freud acknowledged the influence of nine writers who had influenced him greatly. These were the growing band of 'sexologists' who were attempting to unravel the mystery of sex from its cocoon of myth sin and guilt and get to its essential nature. Among these writers were Krafft-Ebing whose 'Psychopathia Sexualis' brought the pervert into the light of day. His (and Magnus Hirschfeld's) work spawned a vast amount of publications on homsexuality and was instrumental in one of the other acknowlegee, Havelock Ellis, to enquire into the meaning and practice of 'normality'.

Havelock Ellis was a man of his time and as such his 'science' like all science is not neutral, it was embedded in and reflected the culture of the day. His book 'Man and Woman' (1894) details the primary, secondary and tertiary characteristics of men and women and is written in a lyrical, populist, romantic style. The major feature of his work is the reinforcement, if not the invention of the concept of 'normality' as being heterosexual. Most of the scientific research on differences between the sexes has consciously or unconsciously been influenced by social values, but the danger in this particular work was for social problems to be recast as theoretical certainties. By defining normality so precisely and ensuring that the male drive was seen as an overwhelming drive with as its object the female, it put two groups in society - females and homosexuals - at a distinct disadvantage. If one has a norm, then by definition anything that does not conform is deviant or perverse and so female sexuality unless passive and/or male-directed is seen in a similar light to male homosexuality as a perversion. Ellis's views were embraced by the rising medical profession and as such given respectability to the stereotyped attitudes to women. Some members went even further by actually presenting case studies to support the concept of female sexuality as hysterical, weak and requiring anti-abortion and birth control legislation. Even a reformer such as Marie Stopes took on board Ellis's ideas and led her to consider women deprived of regular coitus as literally sex starved and indeed for perfect health they should only have orgasms by their husbands.

It was the sexual anaesthesia that Ellis attributed to women that caused the rise of so many volumes on the frigidity of women in the 1920s. Frigidity had many faces. At its most simplistic it was defined as an aversion to sexual intercourse or failure to reach orgasm. This was hardly surprising as the current thinking was that orgasm was reached via the penis in the vagina, despite the amount of anecdotal evidence provided to Marie Stopes (Caplan, 1992), such as, 'Doctor, have I got to put up with this? I can't bear it pumping in and out'. Women again were the losers in this discourse, for not only were they not brought to orgasm by the man, it had to be their fault. For frigidity was not merely seen as absence of orgasm or pleasure in sex, it was seen as an act of resistance against the man. It could not be his inexperience, lack of finesse or simple boorishness, because according to Ellis she had to be willing to have an orgasm, and much of the courtship he advocated was a means to the end of overcoming this `resistance'.

The difficulty for women with the concept of frigidity, as so many feminist writers have pointed out is that although women were now allowed to have sexual feelings, and did not merely, as in Victorian times, have to lie back and think of England, they did need a man to be fulfilled. This was at a time that female emancipation was a big issue and they were beginning to achieve a measure of independence. What this concept did was to rein in female sexuality and take away any autonomy from women. A woman had to be sexually passive and dependent on a man for arousal, a 'sleeping princess' in truth. A whole schema for women emerged from frigidity. As female sexuality could not exist without men there were the true women who enjoyed intercourse with their husband and posed no threat to the supremacy of the male. There were frigid women who, by actively resisting men, were a challenge to masculine authority and needed to accept the facts of life, and there was a third type, the lesbian. These were a mystery to men as their sexuality did not need awakening by a man so they couldn't be 'real' women. They were explained away as being so inverted that they formed a third, masculine-type gender and not being women they posed no threat to men. There was another anomaly in this discourse and that was the existence of the female instinct. If as Freud said, the instinct was an everpresent and driving force then the notion of a female instinct that can only be awakened by men requires explaining.

From the beginning of the struggle for female emancipation women have attempted to make visible the extent to which human sexuality has been defined by men as subject and experienced by women as object. In the early years of suffrage there was a measure of male support for their political activities. However in the 1960s and early '70s with the rise of the women's liberation movement, which highlighted more acutely the masculinization of human sexuality, the 'sisters' found themselves alone. They started to challenge the assumptions on all levels and when they commenced with the male notions of sexual beauty and pleasure found themselves harangued and vilified as dykes and sags. Although there was a large measure of support from 'ordinary' women there were confusions and divisions which according to Margaret Jackson (1991), were directly or indirectly attributable to the interventions of science and medicine into the sexual-political arena. The three main advances that the feminist movement had to make were, first a self-recognition, i.e. an identification with other women, or a certainty of approach. The second advance was probably the most difficult, and that was a theoretical framework for the construction of a satisfactory female femininity, and thirdly a way of living a personal or individual life that supported the theoretical politics. Obviously as all women in Western society have been subtly influenced by the 'penis envy' or female genital inferiority it was and is not (for it is still continuing) an easy road to travel. This is particularly so when an endeavour is made to reconcile the two arms of the movement, i.e. female heterosexuality and lesbianism. The politics of feminist ideology have homed in on the conjunction of male sexuality and power and out of this has come a raising of the public's awareness of such issues as biological sex and political awareness, male violence, particularly that of rape, pornography and child sexual abuse. The discussion has been on-going since the 1970s, and although at times the diversity of opinion has been divisive and frustrating to any single coherent agreed thinking on feminism, what it has done is to air the topic of female sexuality and to generate further debate. Such debate encompasses sexual politics and the reduction of female oppression. It emphasizes the right of women to be sexual in a way that is not defined by men and to self-determination over their own bodies in matters such as contraception and abortion.

A useful aid to the feminist cause was the work of Kinsey (1991) and Masters and Johnson (1966). In 1941 the Association of Women Students at Indiana University in the United States asked for a course in human sexuality for students who were or were about to be married. At that time accurate information on sexual matters was hard to obtain in America. The university asked an eminent zoologist Dr Alfred C. Kinsey to coordinate the course and so a modern day sexologist began his work. What is little known about Kinsey is that he was a credible scientist with over 20 years of study into the anatomy and physiology of gall wasps behind him before he started his work on sexuality. On attempting to develop the curriculum, Kinsey found that there was precious little in the way of researched facts to present to his students and so he began to collect his own data. Eventually he managed to attract funding from the Rockefeller Foundation and with it established the Institute for Sex Research as a non-profit making venture. Kinsey's intentions were to study human sexual behaviour from a non-political, non-legal and non-religious viewpoint and to provide scientific and research-based facts from which individuals could make informed decisions. His was, in effect, a researcher of desire and because it was taken out of the social arena then it lost any religious or moral overtones and everything became natural. So nothing was 'normal' and nothing 'abnormal'. Everything was accepted, collated and analysed and in so doing he revealed interesting facts about male sexuality, the prevalence of homosexuality and the 'activeness' of women. His radical empiricism also challenged phallocentricism.

In 1948 he published his first book, *Sexual Behaviour in the Human Male*, which contained data collated from over 5,000 males. This book was originally intended to cater for the medical profession but became an overnight best seller. Two interesting facts that would have confounded the Victorian moralists were that over 90 per cent of the men masturbated regularly and more than 33 per cent had had a sexual encounter with another man during their adult life. Later on in 1953, *Sexual Behaviour in the Human Female* was published and again the moralists were to be confounded. At least half of the women were not virgins on marriage in an age when virginity was extremely prized in a bride. Women were also found not to be monogamous, at least 25 per cent were involved in extramarital affairs. As these findings challenged the status quo as well as the myth of women's passivity in sexual matters, Kinsey soon found himself in hot water. He was in fact brought before a McCarthy investigatory committee and lost his financial support from the Rockefeller Foundation. Although he died in 1956 the Kinsey institute did and still does continue and has conducted research on a wide variety of topics such as pregnancy and abortion (Kinsey Institute, 1958) and sex offenders (Kinsey Institute, 1965).

Kinsey's work was to inform the body of literature in a way that had not hitherto been done but it was mainly a report of sexual practices and as such provided an invaluable baseline of sociological information. More than that it paved the way for further research into the subject and metaphorically opened the door for other researchers to pass through. One of these was William Masters, a young physician, who with his partner Virginia Johnson was to undertake empirical studies into the nature of the sexual response. They considered that it was impossible to treat patients for sexual inadequacy without first understanding the physiological and psychological responses to sexual stimulation. They conducted detailed observational studies in laboratory settings of the gross physical changes which take place in the male and the female sexual response cycle. They were intent on an accurate and unbiased interpretation of the data and to this end filmed much of their work in colour. This was, of course, not without its difficulties, one of which was the research population itself. There is a possibility that people who are willing to serve as subjects, be artificially stimulated and filmed, may be atypical in their responses. There is also the possibility that the artificial setting may alter the physiology as well as the psychology of the subject. In the event, the population sample was mainly from the upper socioeconomic and intellectual strata of a large university hospital complex (Masters and Johnson, 1966). Their research provided the foundation for much of the information available today (and described in Chapter 4) on the physiology of the sexual response. Masters and Johnson were instrumental in laying the foundations for sex therapists to practice their profession. For example, they dispelled the myth of the danger of masturbation and went further advocating that women should be taught how to masturbate as a means of learning about the rhythms of their own bodies as a precursor to orgasm with a partner.

Another researcher to follow in Kinsey's footsteps was Shere Hite who tackled the issue from yet another angle. She is interested in the quantification and analysis of attitudes and emotions, a very difficult task. She resisted doing this with small samples and emulated Kinsey in his use of a large population sample. She allows the person to speak freely without predefinitions and has published her findings in three monumental books (Hite, 1976, 1984; 1991). Although Hite can be criticized for the flaws in her methodology - for example she has not used a random sampling technique - it must be acknowledged that she has contributed a great deal to the fund of knowledge.

Following this brief overview of the work of the theorists, it is perhaps a good idea to turn to sexuality as praxis. Sexuality is a lived experience and as such is experienced through the senses. As human beings develop within the world they are part of the world in a reflexive sense. As Brake (1982) says, 'we develop through our perceptions, cognitions and understanding of our relationship to the world and to others within it. They are reflected back and mediated by our emotions'. If this is so then human sexuality must be the ultimate in praxis as it is through feelings, attitudes, desires, lusts, loves and envies that we experience sexuality. Self is the subject and the Other is the object in a world where reality is shaped by one's perceptions of it, and they, in turn, are shaped by knowledge received through the senses. As the person develops sexually the self is itself developed and mediated by others. Sexual identity develops, is confirmed and matures in conjunction with the relationship to other people. It does not exist alone, and for its development there has to be a loosening of restraints and a movement towards sexual freedom. This can only happen in a world where one can not only struggle free of one's own repressions, but not be responsible for the oppression of others. This is not easy for, as the theorists and thinkers have shown, if it is as subject-object that one finds gratification in sexual practice then someone has to be Other. According to Beauvoir (1975), the supreme Other in this objectification process is always the woman. To Beauvoir the man-woman relationship is not one of inter subject recipricosity, it is one of female psychic oppression. It is not her body in a biological fashion that is the object but rather it is that she has been alienated and denied her own sexuality and in so doing becomes the second sex.

If this is the case then it is not an intrinsic biological feature that makes for a sexual identity but rather the interpretations and meanings that one gives to the everyday interactions. Sexual identity can then be considered to be mediated through symbols, and behaviour is scripted (Berne, 1968; Gagnon and Simon, 1973). The penis in particular becomes a symbol, the phallus, that extends into all aspects of life e.g. architecture, and what it signifies is man's potency and man's power. Language is another powerful symbolic force and so it is strong, Lacan (1977) would have us believe that it forms the mechanism for a prestructured subjectivity, i.e. the child enters the world of symbolism (language) just when he is at the Oedipal stage.

Likewise, behaviour is scripted as part of the games people play, and the rules are well understood by the actors. They are learned and reinforced over a long period of time and sexual arousal is dependent on the game and the individual's understanding of it. Not only their understanding but their position in the power hierarchy (power as Foucault (1978) points out is always an ingredient will also play a part in the arousal process). For some, being dominant is the only way they can be aroused and for others it is the reverse. Sex then becomes not just a means of reproduction or a source of harmless pleasure, being inextricably linked to power it is capable of being abused and causing abuse. As power is created in the relations that sustain it, or as Berne would say, the game can only go on whilst the actors play it, it also creates the relationships. Foucault suggests that linking the practices and techniques of sex are four types of human subject: the hysterical woman, the masturbating child, the Malthusian couple and the perverse adult. If it is true that the power relations define the sexuality of the body, and society categorizes them, then as sex is seen as a means of access to the life of the body and life of the species, so sex must be a crucial target of power. The categories will then be perpetuated and be regulated or 'normalized' in whatever direction society thinks fit. Individuals' sexual responses may be physiologically similar but they will be socially conditioned to operate.

PART TWO

Sexuality in Practice

CHAPTER FOUR

The Expressive Body

To our bodies turn we then, that so
Weak men on love revealed may look;
Love's mysteries in souls do grow,
But yet the body is his book.

John Donne. (1571-1631) The Ecstasy

Everyone is capable of sexual arousal in one way or another but how it is manifest (or not as the case may be) is, as was discussed previously, dependent on may things such as culture, historical context and socialization. However, physically, there are similarities in the physiological changes such as blood pressure, heart rate, glandular secretions and muscular contractions that make it worthwhile to look at the anatomy of the sex organs and their physiological function in the arousal process.

The female external genitalia (or vulva) contain the labia majora, the labia minora, the clitoris, the vaginal orifice, the urethral orifice, Bartholin's glands and the perineum. Superior to the vulva and lying over the pubic bones is a pad of fat, the Mons veneris or Mount of Venus which is covered by pubic hair growing in a triangular distribution.

The Labia Majora are two thick folds of skin containing a large amount of fatty tissue and a small amount of smooth muscle. Pubic hair grows on the lateral surfaces and both the lateral and medial surfaces contain a large number of sebaceous glands.

The Labia Minora are two thin folds of skin lying just inside the labia majora which merge superiorly to enclose the clitoris in a hood-like fashion. This hood is termed the prepuce. The labia minora contain a vast number of nerve endings and a rich blood supply and in consequence are extremely sensitive to touch. Their surface is composed of stratified squamous epithelium and it contains a great number of sebaceous glands.

The clitoris is a small barrel shaped organ situated within the prepuce at the point where the labia minora meet. It is made up of two small erectile cavernous bodies and ends in a glans or head. It is similar in structure to the penis being made up of erectile tissue and richly endowed with nerve endings and plays an essential role in sexual excitement.

The urethral orifice lies just below the shaft of the clitoris in the midline and is enclosed by the external urethral sphincter. In females it has no other function than to allow the passage of urine.

The vaginal orifice lies below the urethral orifice and is surrounded and enclosed by a sphincter muscle, the bulbo cavernosus. In the virgin it is partially covered by a thin membrane, the hymen, which, after intercourse or the use of tampons, is broken leaving residual tags. Although many cultures lay great store on the presence or otherwise of the hymen it does not seem to have a physiological function.

Inferiorly and laterally on either side of the vaginal orifice lie the greater vestibular or Bartholin's glands. They do not produce a great deal of secretions even during coitus but what secretions there are, are thought to reduce vaginal acidity and increase sperm longevity (Masters and Johnson, 1966).

Connecting the lower part of the vaginal orifice, the introitus, and the anal sphincter is an area of skin, the perineum, which lies over the perineal body and is made up of muscle layers, the transverse perineii, and the pubo coccygeus muscle.

The female internal reproductive organs consist of the vagina, the cervix (the lower third of the uterus), the body of the uterus, the fallopian tubes and the ovaries.

The vagina is a muscular tube approximately 10cm long on its posterior wall and 7.5cm long on the anterior due to the protrusion into the upper aspect of the cervix. Its walls lie in apposition making it a potential rather than an actual tube. The vaginal walls are thrown into folds, rugae, and are lined with mucosa. The vagina itself does not secrete fluid but is lubricated by transudation of lymph from the underlying rich vascular bed. The ph of the vagina is acid, which although hostile to sperm does protect against infection.

The uterus or womb is a muscular pear shaped organ approximately 7.5cm by 5cm by 2.5cm made up of three layers of muscle, the perimetrium (outer), the myometrium (middle) and the endometrium (the inner). It is anteverted and anteflexed and inferiorly its lower third, the cervix, protrudes into the vagina. The Fallopian tubes join the uterus laterally and superiorly at the cornua of the fundus. Under hormonal influence (oestrogen and progesterone) the endometrium thickens each month in preparation to receive a fertilized ovum. In the absence of pregnancy the lining is shed as the menses and the cycle begins again.

The Fallopian tubes lead from the ovaries to the uterus and are responsible for the transportation and nourishment of the ovum. Fertilization occurs in the Fallopian tubes and the fertilized ovum reaches the uterus approximately seven days later. Their lining is of ciliated endothelium, the cilia or fine hairs of which waft the ovum along. At the end nearest the uterus each tube has finger-like endings, the fimbria which move across the ovary at the time of ovulation and sweep the newly released ovum into the fallopian tube.

The ovaries are the primary sex organs of the female and are oval and grey white in colour. They are approximately 3 cm by 2 cm by 1 cm in size and are situated in the pelvis, laterally to the uterus and outside the peritoneum or broad ligament. They are held in position by several ligaments including the ovarian ligament and the suspensory ligament. The surface of the ovary is made up of a modified germinal epithelium which is under hormonal influence and which lies over a fibrous connective tissue layer, the tunica albuginea. The ovary itself is divided into two: an inner medulla containing blood vessels, lymph and nerves and an outer cortex. The cortex contains approximately 400,000 primordial follicles or undeveloped ova. From puberty until the menopause one follicle a month matures and is released from the surface of the ovary.

The breasts are technically not sex glands in that their function is to provide nourishment for the infant. However they do play a part in arousal and in many cultures have an erotic significance. They are two glands that are situated on the anterior chest wall and extend from the first to the fifth rib. They lie over the pectoralis major muscle and are composed of glandular and adipose tissue and are roughly hemispherical in shape with a small amount of tissue extending into the axilla (the axillary tail of Spence). The shape varies from woman to woman and changes over the individual's life span becoming more pendulous and less firm with age. Milk is produced in the lactating female by the glandular tissue and is transported to the outside of the body by a duct and tubule system. The internal duct system leads to openings on the surface of the breast at the nipple. The nipples are composed of erectile tissue and smooth muscle fibres which contain many nerve endings and so the nipple is sensitive to touch and will become erect when the female is sexually aroused.

The male external genitalia consists of the penis, the perineum and the scrotum which contains the testes.

The penis is of variable size particularly in the unaroused state and this does not seem to have an effect on function except perhaps psychologically, as many men (if not all) seem to be obsessed by its size. It consists of erectile tissue arranged in three cylindrical bodies and is covered with a fibrous coat the tunica albuginea and enclosed in thick fascia. The cylindrical bodies are a pair of corpora cavernosa and a corpus spongiosum which contains the urethra. The erectile tissue is a mass of spongelike material which is interlaced with arteries and veins. The distal portion is the head or glans penis formed from the expanded corpus spongiosum. At the base of the penis the corpora cavernosa diverge to form the crura which are firmly attached to the pubic bones. The blood supply is from the internal pudendal arteries. The penis is covered by a covering of skin which is loosely attached at the glans and hangs over to form the foreskin or prepuce.

The scrotum is a sac containing the testes which is made up of a thin layer of skin containing involuntary muscle fibres. During cold weather the scrotum is drawn up to bring the testes into contact with the body and in warmer weather it relaxes causing them to hang further away. This is a regulatory mechanism that protects the function of spermatogenesis which is temperature sensitive.

The male perineum is the area which extends from the symphysis pubis anteriorly to the coccyx posteriorly and laterally from the ischial tuberosities. It can be divided into two triangles, the anterior is called the urogenital triangle and the posterior, the anal triangle.

Male breasts are much less developed than the female and do not produce milk, but the nipple can be very sensitive to the touch and may also play a part in sexual arousal.

The internal male genitalia are made up of the testes, the epididymis, the vas (ductus) deferens, the seminal vesicles, the prostate gland and the bulbourethral (Cowper's) glands.

The testes are the organs of spermatogenesis and are two oval structures each covered with a layer of connective tissue, the tunica albuginea. Internally each testis is divided into compartments which contain highly convoluted seminal tubules. The process of spermatogenesis occurs within the tubules and they contain gametes at various stages of development. The gametes develop into spermatozoa and travel via a short straight tube - the tubulus rectus - into the efferent ducts and from there into the epididymis.

The epididymis are situated within the scrotum and are attached posteriorly to each testis. Each consists of a coiled tube that receives the spermatozoa and, similarly to the Fallopian tubes of the female, is lined with a ciliated columnar epithelium . The cilia are non-motile and are called stereocilia, the function of which is to transport nourishment from the walls of the epididymis to the spermatozoa. The epididymis becomes continuous with the vas deferens at its lower end.

The vas deferens are the continuations of the epididymis and is a smooth tube which ascends up through the scrotum and into the body via the inguinal canal. It is enclosed, along with the nerves and blood vessels in a sheath of fascia, the spermatic cord. The veins returning from the scrotum carry blood at a lower temperature than body heat and are thought to protect the spermatozoa during their journey within the body. The vas deferens run under the peritoneum along the side walls of the peritoneal cavity, cross the ureters and then journey under the bladder where they enlarge to form ampullae. They are joined at this point by the ducts from the seminal vesicles and form a short vessel, the ejaculatory duct, which passes through the prostate gland and enters the urethra.

The seminal vesicles are two sacs of membrane lying laterally to the vas deferens. They produce secretions which contribute to the formation of the seminal fluid which enable the spermatozoa to be propelled along and through the ejaculatory duct. These secretions make up approximately 60 per cent of the seminal fluid and are composed of fructose and prostaglandins. (Interestingly prostaglandins have the effect on the pregnant cervix at term of making it more amenable to oxytocin, thus coitus will provide a natural aid to the commencement of labour.)

The prostate gland is located directly adjacent to the anterior wall of the rectum and is a gland composed of 30-40 tubulo-alveolar glands which secrete a thin, milky fluid which with the secretions from the seminal vesicles make up the seminal fluid.

The bulbourethral glands (Cowper's glands) are two small glands situated at either side of the urethra and they in turn add to the seminal fluid.

Sexual arousal is difficult to define precisely but has been likened to hunger (Bancroft, Myerscough and Schmidt, 1983) in that a hungry person experiences a subjective state which motivates him to find food (Freud's instinct). Accompanying this subjective state are physiological changes such as a drop in the blood sugar (hypoglycaemia) but there are also factors such as the time of day, that cause a conditioned response and this is the case with the sexual response.

Sexual arousal in both male and female can be triggered off in a great many ways and by a variety of stimuli, both physical and psychological. For example, a man's excitement may be triggered at any hour of the day or night by the sight or touch of certain person or things, by certain smells or sounds, or simply by some thoughts, recollections, or fantasies (Haeberle, 1983). These can vary in various people from what might seem the obvious e.g. sight or smell of the opposite sex, to something apparently unconnected, such as a rubber wellington boot. Although all the senses can be involved in the arousal process the sense of touch is probably the one that is most often responsible for sexual arousal. As was shown earlier there are particular areas of the body which are plentifully supplied with nerve endings and extremely responsive to stroking, licking, rubbing and kissing. These are known as the erogenous zones and in the main are the glans penis of the male, the clitoris of the female and the labia minora, the perineum, the anus, the inner thighs, the nipples, the mouth, the neck, the ankles and really just about any area on the body. What is important is the previous experience and the circumstances under which the body is touched. It is highly unlikely that having one's ears syringed will provoke a sexual response, although it not unknown for enemata to be used for such a purpose. Likewise he or she may be sexually aroused through the other senses, for example a piece of music or a smell. Humans give off body odours called pheremones which play a role in sexual stimulation. They do play a part in sexual attraction but what turns one person on will not necessarily have the same effect on another, so just as candlelight, music by Tchaikovsky and red wine may do it for one couple, for another it may be pounding rock music, disco lights and cider. For others it may be the smell of Chanel No 5 perfume or Kouros aftershave, and for others it is more than enough to smell their partner's body especially immediately after exercise. Dependent on the internal readiness of a person and the memories associated with the stimuli is the amount of receptivity. With a high level of receptivity it is unnecessary to have a lengthy period of stimulus and the opposite is true to the extent that unpleasant experiences will cause a negative effect and sexual excitement will be difficult if impossible to achieve, e.g. after rape.

Masters and Johnson (1966) described the human sexual response pattern as a cycle having four phases: excitement, plateau, orgasm and the resolution phase. The first and last phases consume most of the time spent in the response cycle. Sexual excitement may come upon a man suddenly particularly in the adolescent male, but as he grows older and more experienced it will last longer. The primary sign of male excitement is the erection of the penis. As he is stimulated the spongelike structures in the corpora cavernosa and the corpus spongiosum fill with blood and cause the penis under hydraulic pressure to rise and stiffen. Simultaneously the dartos muscle of the scrotum and the spermatic cord contracts causing the testes to be drawn up towards the body. This is also termed penile tumescence and may last from seconds to minutes depending on the individual circumstances. As the excitement increases there is a rise in the heart rate and blood pressure and in fair-skinned men there may appear a flush or red rash over the lower abdomen, the shoulders the neck and the face. The nipples also undergo a change and they become erect towards the end of the excitement phase.

Following full erection the penis may undergo slightly more vasocongestion and the diameter of the shaft will increase. This is the plateau phase and is really nothing more than a continuation of the excitement phase. Cowper's glands may secrete a drop or two of fluid which will be released from the glans penis (which is now a deeper red mottled colour due to venous stasis). They may contain spermatozoa and may well have been and may well be in the future the cause of unplanned pregnancies.

As the myotonia and nervous tension increase there is a sudden peak of tension followed by an involuntary explosive discharge of tension, which causes an instant release followed by a series of involuntary contractions aided by thrusting movements from the pelvis. This is the orgasm which also causes involuntary rhythmic contractions of the internal organs. At first there are about three or four very forceful contractions within a second and they then die away becoming weaker at longer intervals. During the orgasmic phase about a teaspoon of semen is forced out in quick spurts through the urethral orifice. During orgasm not only the penis and the internal genitalia contract. The muscles of the face and various parts of the body including the anal sphincter may be involved as well. Breathing becomes very rapid and the heart and blood pressure rise even further than before. Orgasm and ejaculation usually but not necessarily occur together. Occasionally semen is not forced out under pressure but seeps out after the orgasm as an emission, and sometimes, especially in young boys or in men who have a repeated orgasm very quickly after the first, there may be orgasm without ejaculation at all. In certain other instances the semen is not ejaculated out of the body but is passed into the bladder and later is excreted from the body with the urine.

Following orgasm is the fourth and final phase of the cycle, the resolution phase. This is the period which roughly correlates in length of time to the period of excitement and during which the penis may retain some firmness, but eventually returns to its flaccid state and the rest of the body and the blood pressure return to their unexcited state. Accompanying the physiological resolution is a period of subjective calm. At the beginning of this time, which can last as little as a few minutes in young men and extend into hours for older men,the man is incapable of having another orgasm. This refractory period is thought to be a peculiarly male phenomenon for women are capable of being multi-orgasmic in a short period of time (Masters and Johnson, 1966). Immediately after ejaculation many men start to perspire. This seems to be independent of the amount of physical exertion or the presence of a sex flush. It is usually confined to the hands and feet but may appear on the body.

There is a myth that women are slower to respond to sexual stimulation than males but women vary and some women are quite capable of reaching orgasm within a few seconds of stimulation (Diamond, Diamond and Mast, 1972). There is also the problem that started with Freud's assumption that women who require clitoral stimulation are immature, i.e. they have failed to transfer to vaginal stimulation maturity. However this seems to be all but resolved now with the work of Kinsey and Masters and Johnson confirming what the feminists have long been saying, which is that the vaginal walls are relatively insensitive to touch and for a woman the clitoris is the primary site of the orgasm. In females the first obvious sign of sexual stimulation is wetness of the vagina. The blood vessels surrounding the vagina, the vestibular bulbs, are linked to the clitoris and as the clitoris is stimulated the blood vessels become engorged. Lymph is transuded across the vaginal walls and the whole of the vagina is lubricated. It increases in length and width at the inner end. Sometimes damage caused during childbirth particularly from a large and enthusiastically performed episiotomy can cause interference with this process and cause sexual problems for the woman that are physical, but not, as has often been believed in the past, psychosexual. The clitoris itself undergoes tumescence similarly to the penis, but unlike the penis does not undergo erection. The shaft of the clitoris enlarges to lie in closer apposition to the underlying tissue and retracts further under the prepuce. The labia minora increase to 'a minimum of twice their unstimulated size' (Masters and Johnson, 1966) and become darker in colour. The labia majora flatten out and expose the vaginal orifice, more so in a parous woman.

The whole breast during this phase becomes engorged and swollen, and the nipples become erect and may be elongated by up to 1 cm in length. Most women exhibit the sexual flush on the abdomen, shoulders, neck and face and when orgasm is imminent it can extend to the under surface of the breasts. It may even spread over the thighs, buttocks and the back (it reaches its peak during the plateau period and resolves abruptly during resolution.

The plateau period indicates the time when the excitement has reached a high just prior to orgasm when the clitoris retracts under the prepuce. The outer third of the vagina contracts and Bartholin's glands secrete a few drops of fluid. (Both of these processes can be affected following trauma in labour, and a badly or unsutured tear or episiotomy.) Hyperventilation occurs, the heart rate and the blood pressure having increased. The breasts show their greatest expansion during this phase. Voluntary and involuntary myotonia occurs throughout the body and can be noticed in the hands by the exhibition of involuntary clutching movements.

Just prior to orgasm there is an increase in muscle tension throughout the body and this can be observed by the grimaces of the face and the clutching of the partner by the legs and hands. The buttocks very often contract violently and if the woman is in a supine position she may well elevate her pelvis in thrusting movements. As the orgasm takes place contractions start in the outer third of the vagina (the orgasmic platform). They may be short with a short intercontractile time span (e.g. 0.8 seconds) or they may last longer with correspondingly longer intervals between. Involuntary spans occur in the anal sphincter and the uterus also starts to contract, beginning at the fundus and ending in the lower segment (just as the contractions of labour do). Pregnancy increases sensitivity to the effects of orgasm particularly in the last two trimesters, and in the third trimester has been associated with tonicity. Obviously it can be seen that an orgasmic experience at term may induce labour. The external urethral sphincter may contract in some women but not all and the breasts show no change in this phase except that rapid decongestion of the areolar tissue occurs immediately afterwards and is external evidence that orgasm has been reached.

The blood pressure and heart rate peak and there is often hyperventilation. Women unlike men are very often multi-orgasmic and can rapidly return to orgasm after orgasm. Some women act as if they are having one long orgasm but, according to Masters and Johnson who termed this status orgasms, they are actually having orgasm after orgasm with very short intervals between and accompanied by an advanced baseline of plateau tension.

After the final orgasm the sex organs return to their unexcited state. Their is a loss of tumescence in the breasts and the vagina. The ballooning effect on the vagina disappears and the flush fades. The clitoris re-emerges from the prepuce and the labia minora and majora assume their former shape and size. The heart rate, blood pressure and breathing return to normal. Most women during this phase will find themselves covered by a fine film of perspiration over the back, thighs and anterior chest wall. It appears immediately post-orgasm as a result of the resolution of the vasocongestion which causes the sex flush. This phase is accompanied by deep muscle relaxation and when sleep follows it has been shown to be of the deep, rapid eye movement type. It could be that the relaxation is nature's way of ensuring procreation as the woman may remain on her back with the cervix bathed in seminal fluid.

Having said that the erogenous zones are responsive to a variety of stimuli, it comes as no surprise to learn that a variety of stimulants are used and the object may vary. The religious, legal and medical authorities have all laid down 'norms' for people's behaviours and although they very often do not agree, what they do is to make people believe that there is a way of behaving sexually that is normal and or desirable. Other behaviours which fall outside these prescribed may be termed sinful, immoral, deviant, perverse or illegal. What cannot be said is that they are generally abnormal, for as Kinsey has shown the sexual practices of males and females vary to a considerable degree. As heterosexual contact between adults leads to reproduction and perpetuation of the species it is most often held up to be the natural method of sexual expression. However there are two other means which are favoured by a huge number of people (Reinisch and Beasley, 1990) and they are self- and homosexual stimulation (Chapter 12).

Heterosexual contact is commonly called intercourse, which is a euphemism for coitus, where the penis is inserted in the vagina. This may be true for a majority of heterosexual couples for the majority of the time but it is not true for all, and for some (in the case of certain injury, for example) it may never be true. It is probably better to call heterosexual intercourse any contact between a man and a woman that gives sexual pleasure or causes sexual arousal (Comfort, 1987). Generally speaking this contact falls into four types, which are manual, oral, genital or anal intercourse.

Manual stimulation of each other' genitals plays a major part for many couples. For some it is part of foreplay with the man or the woman touching, stroking and massaging the clitoris and or penis as a prelude to penile penetration. At other times (dependent on the mood or the position) it may be that the stimulation continues throughout. Or the woman may be brought to a multi-orgasmic state by masturbation of the clitoris prior to the man's orgasm. The combinations are endless and give rise to the fun of trying. Touching, stroking and caressing are very often afterplay when the object is not sexual arousal as a means of showing affection.

Men or women may lick, kiss or suck the other's genitalia. When the male is the recipient it is termed fellatio and when the woman it is cunnilingus. As with manual stimulation they can be performed as a prelude or as the total experience itself and it is extremely effective in stimulating the sensitive clitoris in a non-aggressive way. According to Kinsey, more than 90 per cent of married couples have engaged in oral sex. It is a very variable practice in that some women will fellate their partner to the point of orgasm but will not allow it to take place in their mouths, whereas other women are reported to enjoy the taste of semen. There is no evidence that sperm itself is harmful unless the man has a sexually transmittable disease such as syphilis or carries the AIDS virus or is positive for Hepatitis B. If this is the case contact should be avoided or a condom used. Some authorities advocate caution in the use of cunnilingus in pregnancy. There is thought to be a small risk of air being blown into the uterus and causing an air embolus. There are no recorded cases in this country since the the commencement of publication of the *Confidential Enquiries into Maternal Deaths* (HMSO, 1952-1990) of such an embolus forming. Another factor which may mitigate against such a happening is the presence of the operculum or thick mucous plug which seals the cervix in pregnancy.

Many couples like the smell of each other and oral genital sex enhances that pleasure. It may be performed in any position but one that is often reported is the 69 position where both partners engage in it at the same time, each with his or her mouth on the other's sex organs.

Genital intercourse has been thought to be the only natural method of intercourse in this country for many centuries. It is probably still true to say that a majority of people indulge in heterosexual genital sex, but how and how often is still unknown. According to Kinsey the most popular position in the West is the missionary position, so-called Pacific islanders are reputed to term it such as it varied from their own preferred woman on top position. In this position the partners face each other with the woman lying on her back with the man between her legs. There are a great many other positions, for example with the man and woman both facing the same way where the penis enters from behind, or with the woman lying or sitting on top of the supine man. In fact the only limit to the number of positions is the agility and imagination of the couple. It may be worth noting here that the penis does not have to be fully inserted into the vagina for semen to be released and find its way to the ovum. This misconception has lead many young women to get pregnant after heavy petting which they considered as 'safe'.

Anal coitus has been indulged in by 20-40 per cent of married woman according to a study cited by Kinsey. The anus is a highly erogenous zone and this practice is variable. It may mean the insertion of a finger or an object into the man's anus during genital intercourse or it may involve the licking or kissing of each other's anus. Or it may be orgasm reached between the woman's thighs or buttocks or full insertion of the penis into the woman's rectum. It can be performed in many positions such as the woman sitting on the man's knee or lying on her stomach or bending over. The practice is still illegal in this country between a heterosexual couple. It may be quite painful and unpleasant for a woman particularly if she is not happy about the practice. It can also be dangerous if the penis is inserted into the vagina without being washed, for harmful bacteria may enter the vagina or the urethra. The overwhelming danger of this practice in this day and age is obviously the risk of transmission of the AIDS virus. It does have to be pointed out, however, that the practice does not cause the virus to be present, it merely facilitates its transfer, so if neither partner are infected neither can catch it.

Self-stimulation or masturbation was at one time held to be one of the worst practices that anyone could indulge in (see Chapter 1). People were warned of the dire consequences they could expect from such action which included death (from divine judgement based on the sin of Onan, Genesis Ch.38, v.8-10) to madness and blindness (Tissot, in Haeberle, 1983). Well into the 19th century this practice was correlated with insanity and thought to lead to psychopathic behaviour. Habitual masturbators were recommended to be locked up in asylums and parents exhorted to prevent their children, however young, from indulging. This led to babies and small children being put to bed with their hands tied to stop them handling their genitals. However, nowadays it is considered a harmless, universal and beneficial practice. Masters and Johnson recommended the teaching of it as part of sex therapy, and as one wit observed, it is a practice that allows one to meet a nicer class of person. According to Kinsey 94 per cent of males and 40 per cent of females reported having masturbated to orgasm, and may do it more or less frequently during their lifespan, depending on various factors such as libido, or social circumstances and availability of a partner. The only problem that may occur from the practice is becoming dependent on the use of artifacts or special techniques to reach orgasm, which necessitate it and limits the person to that way of sexual expression. Some people have pointed out that the use of pornography in the masturbatory process can have antisocial effects but as yet there is no proven causal relationship.

Just as there is no norm in the West so it is across the world. Sexual practices are as varied as the peoples who practice them. Whatever the practice, there will be some cultures that condem it whilst others praise it. There are no stereotypes for, as was shown in the discussion on gender, the sexual identity of a person will influence his or her social behaviour and what that behaviour is depends on what is valued as culturally acceptable within the context of the individual's social and cultural world.

CHAPTER FIVE

From Cradle to Grave

All the world's a stage,
And all the men and women merely players:
They have their exits and their entrances;
And one man in his time plays many parts,
His acts being seven ages.

Shakespeare (1564-1616)
As You Like It., *Act II, Scene 7*

As Freud pointed out all men (and women) are sexual creatures through-out the whole of the life span, not merely as Shakespeare thought, in the third age as the lover, 'sighing like a furnace, with a woeful ballad made to his mistress' eyebrow' (Shakespeare, c.1600). During the 100 or so years before Freud developed his theory, Britain and the West had moved away from their earlier recognition of the child as a sexual being. Being uncomfortable with their own sexuality was extended to the child, sometimes in a most bizarre fashion (such as having parts of a child's genital tissue surgically removed to prevent `unnatural' hab-its) (Haeberle, 1983). Freudian psychoanalysis was acknowledged as a powerful discourse. Having been taken on board by a large follow-ing it meant that child sexuality had to be acknowledged and exam-ined. This examination proved not to be thorough for his myth of the `latency' period was also believed. This was despite the fact that all people who have the responsibility for the day-to-day care of children will be aware that they demonstrate genital behaviour of a sexual type, such as penile erection, from an early age. They also indulge in some form of sex play throughout childhood. This may take the form of showing each other their genitalia, playing `doctors and nurses' or even indulging in mock coitus. Sex play usually starts at about four or five which is just about the time that Freud maintained that children were entering a latent phase where sexual activities were in abeyance until adulthood.

Babies exhibit penile erection and vaginal lubrication either during their sleep or when they are feeling warm and relaxed, it is very common, for example, during a cuddle or after a bath. These manifestations are unlike adult responses in that they are involuntary responses. As the child matures he or she explores his or her body, sucks the toes and plays with the genitals. Although little boys may have an erection it is unlikely that they will have an orgasm, although babies and children can be capable of so doing (Reinisch and Beasley, 1990). They do not, however, masturbate to orgasm as adults do.

The move from self-play to peer play in childhood is thought to be part of a normal learning continuum that in healthy people develops both their self-esteem and the ability to interact with others (Reinisch and Beasley, 1990). The other determining factor in this equation is parental attitude. Parents transmit their feelings about sexuality to their children in many powerful ways, such as the words they use or do not use to name the genitalia, the attitude they have to their own and the child's nudity. Even the expressions on their faces reveals their values. Most behaviours follow an orderly and continuous sequence but many behavioural psychologists have broken up this process into stages (Burns, 1991) and these are the stages during which, according to Erikson (1963), trust or mistrust and initiative or guilt and industry or inferiority develop. So if the child is taught to be comfortable with his sexuality and is not made to feel guilty then a healthy psychosexual development will occur. Sexuality should be acknowledged and correct information given and misinformation corrected. It is easier and better to give facts as and when necessary, rather than waiting and hoping that they will be given the information by teachers later on. It is highly unlikely that this will happen and they are more likely to be ill-informed by their peers. This again tells the child something of the parents' attitudes. The children may be made to feel guilty and this will impair their future sexual development. There are lots of opportunities and there are lots of aids, such as anatomically correct little boy dolls and pregnant dolls complete with removable fetus.

Adolescence is a relatively new social construction. Not long ago children were born and worked alongside their parents doing what they were physically strong enough to cope with. (This is still true for the vast majority of children on this planet.) In a mining disaster at Leigh in Lancashire in the 1700s, the youngest colliery worker to be killed in the explosion was a three-year-old girl whose job it was to waft air down the pit by pulling on a rope attached to a wooden door. Following puberty the child was considered old enough to marry or at least have sexual relationships (think of Romeo and Juliet who were only in their early teens). Now, however, in this age of extended childhood there is an in-between phase which is socially recognized as adolescence. In many cultures the period of adolescence is extremely short and is the time when puberty is seen to have occurred, e.g. the commencement of the development of secondary sex characteristics such as pubic hair or the menarche in girls. It is followed quite rapidly by an initiation ceremony or rite of passage into man or womanhood (although formal ceremony occurs less frequently for girls than boys). However, in the modern West there are relatively few formal procedures for this process, and even a Jewish boy's Barmitzvah at 13 is more of a token gesture to manhood than a practical reality. Adolescence is the period of time which commences with puberty and lasts until the late teens. It is the period of an individual's life where sexuality is dominated by an emotional see-sawing between ecstasy and agony. The non-conventional adolescent is a rare bird indeed, and what the individual's peer group thinks becomes a matter of major importance and the appearance of a spot is a tragedy. Socially the person is seen as needing a long time to adjust to the realities of adult life and the privileges and rights are bestowed in a fragmentary fashion. For example, an adolescent can legally indulge in heterosexual coitus and can also legally get married at 16 but cannot vote or drink alcohol until the age of 18. Financially, many adolescents are dependent upon their parents for much longer than was the norm in Britain until the 1960s or early '70s. This is due to a combination of factors such as the recession and poor prospects of employment, linked with low wages and poorly-funded training courses. There is a move towards attracting more and more young people into further and higher education which also leaves them impecunious. Traditionally, young people were seen to be adult when they went out to work and/or married. As these may not be viable options any more in socially disadvantaged areas it may account in some degree for the increase in pregnancies to young unmarried teenagers. Could it be that motherhood is a rite of passage into adulthood for a young woman with no prospect in the foreseeable future of having a job or her own home any other way?

Physically, adolescence starts with puberty, which generally occurs between 9 and 11 years of age in girls and 9 and 15 years of age in boys. It begins as a result of hormonal changes but what triggers off the changes is uncertain. In girls, the cyclical production of follicle stimulating hormone, luteinizing hormone, oestrogen and progesterone starts the physical development of the secondary sex characteristics and the commencement of the menstrual cycle and normal vaginal secretions. First, the areola around the nipple enlarges and darkens slightly and then the breasts themselves start to develop. This is followed or accompanied by the growth of pubic and axillary hair which is completed by about the age of 16. Sweat and oil glands become more productive and some girls (but less so than boys) will develop acne. This period is often preceded by a growth spurt, but following the menarche growth seems to slow down with very little increase after the age of 16.

In boys the changes are more subtle and less definitive than they are in girls. The first signs are a growth in size of the testicles and the skin of the scrotum thickens, darkens and pubic hair appears sparsely. Under the effect of increased amounts of testosterone the body starts to develop its male shape. The shoulders and arms develop and the hips appear narrower. Body hair may appear but this is variable between individuals and in some cultures, such as Far Eastern or North American Indian, it is extremely rare. At about 14 years of age the larynx enlarges causing the voice to deepen. This can be a period of great uncertainty for young men, as they never know whether they will produce a deep resonance or a high-pitched squeak. Pubic hair starts to proliferate around this time and the penis enlarges, spermatozoa is produced from anytime from the age of 11 to 17 and nocturnal emissions are common. Facial hair appears anytime from 14 to 19 years depending on the colouring and skin type. Shaving may be necessary once in a while or every day. There is often a great growth spurt during this period which is virtually finished by the age of 18, but muscle development and some increase in height may go on into the 20s.

According to the latest Kinsey report (Reinisch and Beasley, 1990) most adolescent males and a sizeable number of girls engage in self-stimulation. Many boys are taught to masturbate by other boys, but the girls more often learn by themselves. The methods vary from boy to boy and girl to girl but are usually a variation of the penis being rubbed and or inserted into something tubular like a toilet roll holder and the clitoris being rhythmically stimulated by direct rubbing or indirect pressure from caressing the vulva or the legs being squeezed together. It is a time of fantasizing and learning about one's own body and the lessons learned can be used to give pleasure to a partner later on. Sometimes, particularly for boys, visual aids are used such as soft pornographic material.

Homosexual contact can be quite common at this time, particularly for boys, who may indulge in group masturbation, but does not necessarily lead to predominately homosexual behaviour.

Adolescence is a period of searching for answers to questions about who one is, what one's identity really means and it is, on the whole, a period of examining values, beliefs and practices learned in childhood. This is the time that Erikson (1963) considered to be one of 'identity crisis', when old values are challenged, role confusion is strong and alternative lifestyles are appealing. (It is worth mentioning that many studies do not agree with Erikson on this point (Burns, 1991). It is a time of bodily and mental change when physical maturity conflicts with social immaturity to give rise to frustration and anger. This gives rise to mood swings which can be extremely frequent leading to impulsive and aggressive or silly behaviour followed by periods of mature and sensible behaviour.

This can be a stormy period for the family and a time when the young adolescent may indulge in risk-taking such as unprotected sex, as a challenge to the authority of his or her parents, a quest for adventure or simply as a result of peer pressure. This can lead to untimely pregnancies and a risk of sexually transmitted disease such as chlamydia, gonorrhoea, syphilis or even the AIDS complex. Many teenagers even now are ignorant in matters to do with sexual health and contraception and are in need of sex education of a specific and practical kind, such as the provision of information and condoms.

As teenagers become older they tend to have a more balanced view of sexual activity than most previous generations have and are able to talk about sexual matters more easily than ever before. This is not to say that the emotional side of relationships is any less fraught, for it is still a time of self-preoccupation and concerns and sometimes over concerns about the body, its shape size and weight as compared to an imaginary standard. More often than not these concerns revolve around the size of the breasts (are they too big or too small or the wrong shape or unevenly sized?) and the penis (is it too small and why won't it behave?). Occasionally this may be linked to an irrational fear of sexuality which occurs typically in girls and can lead to anorexia with its accompanying amennorhoea and child-like figure.

Despite all the problems, there is, as every parent is glad to be told but doesn't quite believe, life after adolescence. On the positive side the individual becomes calmer and more mature and yet although one wouldn't want to remain on that emotional roller coaster it is a stage that one can remember nostalgically with a sigh for its intensity and passion.

Adulthood is the time from the end of adolescence until the end of life. Towards the end of life as the body starts to age the changes may bring health problems and infirmities that can affect actual or perceived sexual functioning. Before that, however, the most dramatic change that can take place is parenthood.

During the female menstrual cycle there is a point when an ovum that has matured under the influence of follicle stimulating hormone and luteinizing hormone bursts from the surface of the ovum and is wafted into the fallopian tube where it begins its journey to the uterus. The remaining depression on the ovary is a yellowish colour and is called the corpus luteum. The cells of this area produce the hormone progesterone. If the ovum is not fertilized the production of progesterone by the cells of the corpus luteum begins to diminish and by the 14th day the supply is so low that by a feedback mechanism the hypothalamus produces stimulating hormones that cause the pituitary gland to produce follicle stimulating hormone which starts the process again. The lining of the uterus along with the unfertilized ovum is shed as the menses.

Oestrogen produced at this time has an effect on the mucous of the cervix making it more amenable to the passage of spermatozoa. It also seems to have an effect on a woman's readiness for sex. Women do not have a set period of oestrous as mammals do when they are receptive to the advances of the male but it has been reported (Masters and Johnson, 1966) that many women do have an increase in libidinal energy at this time. If coitus takes place there is a good chance that conception will occur. The sperm have to swim upstream through the external cervical os, through the cervical canal into the uterus via the internal cervical os, up the body of the uterus and into the fallopian tubes via the cornuus. This long journey is only managed by the strongest and many do not survive along the way. Once the ovum is reached it is surrounded by spermatozoa, but only one is able to enter and cause fertilization. Once fertilization has occurred the cell wall of the ovum becomes impervious to entry by any other. The fertilized ovum causes a hormone, human gonadotrophic hormone, to be produced. This maintains the corpus luteum and thus ensures a constant supply of progesterone which maintains the pregnancy. At about 14 weeks gestation the developing placenta becomes the major supplier of progesterone and the corpus luteum is relatively redundant.

The fertilized ovum which by now has multiplied into a cluster of cells - the morula - embeds into the rich lining of the uterus and develops and differentiates into the embryo and later the fetus and the placenta.

The pregnancy will last (full-term) 40 weeks, after which the baby will be born either vaginally or by caesarean section. During the pregnancy both men and women will find that they are readjusting their lives. The effect of pregnancy on women is considered a great deal both from the psychological and physiological angles, but there is relatively little written on the effect of pregnancy on men and even less on the effect of pregnancy on the sex lives of men and women. This will be addressed in later chapters and for now there needs to be only mention of the effects on sexuality of being a parent.

In previous chapters the physiology and politics of sexuality were discussed, but there is another aspect of sex in the lives of adult people and that is providing an atmosphere of intimacy and bonding. If people are thought to be mere functioning machines then sex will fall into two camps which may or may not coincide. They are the hedonistic aspect where pleasure is the be all and end all. This may or may not include pleasure for the partner. If it does, then both partners can gain a great deal of joy from the encounters, but if it does not, then it may be a very dangerous road altogether. For as Freud (1986) pointed out, Eros can be coupled with Thanatos to produce sadistic enjoyment of sex, and sadism can never be ethical or justifiable because it involves the abuse of power and the exploitation of a weaker party. The other camp for sex to fall into is for reproduction alone. This (pardon the pun) has to be a sterile route and one that many women in the West in the past had to travel to beget an heir for an otherwise disinterested partner and one that many women the world over may still have to go down to produce children, or those of a particular sex.

However, there is another reason for sex, and according to Bancroft, Myerscough and Schmidt (1989) it is that of strengthening the pair bond or encouraging a couple to stay together. It fosters intimacy and makes life less stressful, there is someone to share worries and fears with and who will be a helpmeet in every sense. It has been found to relieve stress and reduce anxiety. It benefits the pair as a couple and enables personal growth. It is very healthy for couples to be free of constraints in their sex life except those they make themselves. It does not bode well if they are constrained by external factors such as worrying about stereotype behaviour. For example, men need not and perhaps should not always initiate sex, but if a woman (or a man) think that a woman who does take the lead is fast (or any other negative view) then their relationship will be the poorer for it. Likewise if the one or both think that sex is some sort of athletic encounter where performance is measurable against a norm, then they are setting themselves up for unhappiness. As the latest Kinsey report has shown, the variety of human sexual behaviour encompasses such a wide variety of methods and appetites that it is misleading and unhelpful to think of a 'norm'.

Another factor and perhaps the major constraining factor of sexual practice in parents is the presence of their children. It may be that they are physically tired from lack of sleep due to a crying baby or the presence of a toddler who insists on coming into the parental bed at night. Or they may feel obliged to curtail their sexual activities because of the presence of teenagers in the house. It may be that these factors, which might not matter to one couple, would be enough to dampen ardour in one or both of the partners of another couple. This does not mean that they are incapable of being aroused or that they have psychological difficulties, rather it is that they are less than ready. It is up to the pair to decide how to overcome these problems in the best way for themselves. What they should not do is too get so hung up on the irritations that they become problems. For example, many men may fail to achieve or maintain an erection when they are stressed or worried and this can happen particularly when their wives are pregnant or they have just had a baby. There seems to be two ways of handling such a situation. These are for either the man himself or the woman to think he is a failure and to reinforce this with either comments or body language. This will probably lead to self fulfilling behaviour and a continuation of the problem and maybe even a breakdown in the relationship. Or the couple can think of it as it is a transient period in their lives and one in which the solution lies in a temporary change in sexual habits. They may find that if the man concentrates during this time on helping his partner to achieve orgasm, perhaps by clitoral stimulation alone, then the problem will be self-limiting. The only difficulty is that if it happens because the a man is feeling insecure, for example, he may feel displaced in his partner's affections by a new baby then he will need a lot of genuine reassurance of her continued interest. This may pose a problem for couples who are not well versed in sexual matters and one or either thinks that sexual intercourse necessitates male orgasm in the vagina. Therapists suggest that people who have difficulties responding, or who have low sexual desire may be helped by concentrating on a sexual situation or person as an aid to arousal. Or they may need to make time and space for themselves, such as sending the children to the grandparents and having an erotic evening to themselves. A glass of wine, a hot bath, a massage with aromatic oils and a willingness to relax, learn and enjoy each other's company without inhibitions and expectations may help.

As people age they have a gradual drop in circulating hormones which will affect sexual function in one way or another. In women there is only a very gradual reduction of circulating hormones, particularly oestrogen, from about the age of 35 which is accompanied by a dramatic drop in her late 40s, which heralds the menopause and by the average age of 51 most women have had their last menstrual cycle. Ovulation can be irregular for several years before the final cessation of the menses and occasionally can occur several months after the periods have apparently ended. This may result in undesired pregnancy, so it is advisable to continue taking contraceptive measures for at least a year after the last period. When the levels of oestrogen in particular fall there are accompanying changes in some of the body systems. One development is the depletion of the calcium stored in the bones leading to a condition, osteoporosis, which may cause the bones to fracture more easily and lead to shrinkage between the vertebrae and loss of height. There is change in the musculature and nerve supply to the pelvic region leading to a potential loss of uterine, bladder or bowel tone and vaginal dryness. The menopause is not an easy time to generalize about. For some women, particularly in our youth-orientated culture, it is a time of sadness and despair. They may feel depressed at the thought of old age on the horizon and they feel physically unwell. It may be a time when they have lost their partner or are resigned to not having one at all. Some women cannot cope with their biological time clock ticking away and may regret not having children, or they may attempt a last ditch exercise in motherhood. The physical side of sexual relations may not be appealing. For some it is the dryness of the vagina that causes discomfort or for others it is their distaste at viewing their own or their partner's ageing body.

However, it is not all doom and gloom. Some women welcome the menopause and find a new lease of life. They are free from the fear of pregnancy, they may be financially more secure than they were in their earlier years and they may now at last have privacy at home because the children have left home. They may now be very experienced in their sexual behaviour and know what pleases themselves and their partners. It may be that many women are content to maintain their general health with exercise, a good diet, being a non-smoker and using a vaginal lubricant if necessary. Others may feel the need to have hormone replacement therapy to counteract the physical effects of the menopause. Generally speaking, women may need a little more attention to foreplay than they did when they were younger, but they are still capable of having a lengthy excitement phase. There may be a quicker return to the unexcited state but physiologically women are capable of having a good sex life well into their 80s (Masters and

Johnson, 1966). The three main problems for women in old age are lack of a partner, or a male partner who cannot maintain his erection, and stiffness in the joints. Masturbation and a little imagination will help in all cases.

Men do not go through a dramatic change at the end of middle age as women do (but then they did not start dramatically either). As a general rule they continue to produce semen until the end of their days and there are many men who father children in their 80s (Charlie Chaplin and Cary Grant are well-known examples). Men seem only to have a gradual drop in the levels of testosterone produced. This may result in a slower rate of arousal time and they may need direct stimulation of the penis and the erection may not be as hard. They may produce less semen and the number of non-ejaculatory type orgasms may gradually increase. The orgasm itself may not be as forceful, as the muscles lose their tone and as the man becomes older there are an increased number of times when the ejaculate is an emission rather than a forceful expulsion. It may take him a long time to recover and the refractory period which could have been a few minutes in an adolescent may have lengthened to hours.

The difficulty for older people and their ability to express themselves sexually is the attitude of society. There seems to be a thinking that older people should gradually become sexless and those that obviously are not are labelled dirty old men and women. This is quite sad, for men and women in their twilight years can have an active sex life even without a partner. Unfortunately they may be denied the opportunity by the society they live in (elderly people's homes, for example). However, this may be changing now since there is an increasing openness about sexual matters tand health professionals in particular are being taught a holistic approach to care, which in theory means a consideration of the person as a sexual being.

A consideration of the person as a sexual being also means understanding that there is non-erotic sexuality. It has already been pointed out that children can be sexual beings without being erotic and so it can be for any period of life. Sexuality is part of all human life and can be expressed by touching, cuddling or just lying close together. This can be very important for the elderly or those who are ill or dying. In one graphic account of his wife's dying and ultimate death, the author was told by the husband how he just lay stretched out on the bed alongside her, barely touching so as not to cause pain but in communion just the same. Sex does not have to be orgasm directed.

On a lighter note, orgasm is not always possible for all people all of the time, so many fake it. According to one researcher (Darling and Davidson, 1986) 59 per cent of women in a sample population of 745 female nurses admitted to faking orgasm. This is not always believed by men unless - as was spelled out so graphically in the 1989 film , 'When Harry Met Sally' - it is demonstrated in the cold light of day across a restaurant table. The sad fact is, that if people feel the need to fake it there must be two factors at work, orgasm directed behaviour and lack of proper communication between the partners. It may be done out of kindness to spare the others feelings or it may be done out of boredom to speed up the process. Whatever the reason it may be easier in the long run to have a more open communication, which could reduce the likelihood of sex being a bore or unsatisfying for one and the need for the other to always achieve.

Another aspect of sexuality is celibacy. This has been advocated in many of the major world religions sometimes, as was seen in Chapter 1, with devastating results for the practitioners. Islam tends on the whole to be non-ascetic with both heterosexual and homosexual sexuality being viewed as acceptable within certain parameters, e.g. within marriage. In Hinduism (which is not technically a religion, rather an encompassing of spiritual beliefs and practices) there are two ways of viewing sexuality. One is the outlook exemplified in the Sanskrit sutras (aphorisms) such as the Kama Sutra of Vatsyayana which shows that sexuality is not unnatural or condemned by God. This is taken to its furthest point by the Tantric sect who rejected the abstract approach of much of Hinduism and developed a practical approach to spirituality that encompassed ritual sexuality (Fuerstein, 1990). The other view is the one practised by Mahatma Ghandi from the age of 36, that of brahmacharya. This is a philosophy which entails transcending the needs and desires of the body and is achieved in the main by fasting, abstinence and meditation. . Part of this is an attempt to gain control over the sexual organs and the 'vital force' semen which leaves one free to rise above the ego and above kama which Ghandi (1927) and others (Bhaktivedanta Swami Prabhupada AC, 1982) equated with lust or desire. This was sometimes used to justify the protection of women, so if they were to be treated as full human beings and capable of a public life, sex, except for procreation, should be tabooed (Caplan, 1991). This is very possibly yet another face of patriarchy.

CHAPTER SIX

In Face of the Odds

Pit any couple in a knot
They canna lowse and needna try,
And mair o'love they'll ken
-if ocht! - than joy'll alone descry.
MacDiarmid (1892-1978)
The Feminine Principle.

Disability, like gender, motherhood, sexuality and childhood, is a social construct and as such plays a big part in the game of consequences
which is life. Just as the social context determines the characteristics
that are assigned to people of one or the other biological sex, so it
does with those who are deemed disabled. Their experience is within
the social context and influenced by cultural and socioeconomic factors. Disabled people are attributed with certain characteristics that set
them apart from mainstream society such as poverty, loneliness and
stigma (Morris, in Swain *et al*, 1993). They are marginalized in both
social, economic and institutional terms. They are stereotyped as dependent and lacking in autonomy, which in some respects resembles
the stereotype of the child. This is particularly difficult for disabled
men, since Western society perceives the stereotypical man as assertive, even aggressive, active and in charge. Masculinity for a disabled
man can be 'an oppressive construct' (Morris, in Swain *et al*, 1993),
but it may be that he can use his gender to resist the passivity thrust
upon him by the well-meaning. This may be more difficult for disabled women as they have to cope with the dual handicap of their
disability and the social construction of femininity which all women
have to deal with. Passivity is seen to be a part of the female persona
and as such aggressive or assertive woman are acting out of character.
This being so, it can be much more difficult for disabled women to
assert their right to autonomy and independence. Unfortunately the
sense of powerlessness of both men and women with disabilities is
not of their making. It is related to the way that society lays down
norms for people to behave. As work and leisure activities are linked

to the attributed characteristics of gender, so is sexual behaviour and self-image. The norm for disability is that it is 'a personal tragedy needing medical treatment' (Oliver, 1990) and the disabled have become one of the 'other' and excluded from the mainstream of life.

So a disabled person is constructed as tragic, sad, powerless and in need of care and a setting apart. What does that do to a person's self-image? Not a lot, is the gut reaction. Disabled people face a lot of prejudice and in the area of sexuality in particular. All of us are, as Foucault pointed out (in Jacobus, 1990), subject to cultural control over the body which is exercised and dieted into the 'ideal' shape (which can change over time). The successful manage to control their body and are seemingly successful members of society. However it may be that they are actually demonstrating their helplessness to confront the system and be anything other than normalised people within the structure. People who do not conform because they do not choose to, such as the overweight overeater, or cannot, such as the person with a disability face a set of assumptions. For the fat these include being characterized as weak-willed and greedy and for the disabled it includes being thought of as sad, bitter, asexual or sexually inadequate and incapable of normal expressions of sexuality. On the whole this is not true, but there is an issue here, as self-concept is linked to body image and these in turn are linked to libido, desire and arousal. If one is constantly being made to feel that one's body fails to meet the standard requirements then one may lose confidence and develop a poor self-concept. This, in turn, may lead to loss of libido or to the development of psychosexual problems. However it must be emphasized that this is not the norm. What is the norm for disabled people is the number of factors that mitigate against their sexual functioning and these are chiefly social, mental and physical.

Social factors include restrictions on sexual activity imposed by other people such as family or institutions. Parents may have quite an inhibiting effect on the sexual behaviour of their children. It is often hard for a parent to accept the fact that their children are sexually active. It brings with it all sorts of fears. For some it can be a reminder of their own mortality. If one's child is old enough to have a child of his or her own (or actually does have one) then it puts the parent into the next generation and this can be frightening. For others it can be the thought of an unwanted pregnancy or the possibility of their child contracting the AIDS virus that worries them. Most parents get over these feelings and welcome the freedom that comes with having an adult child. However, for the parents of a child with physical or mental disabilities this may not be an option that they feel is open to them. They may be so bound up with the physical care that they give, that they cannot see that their child needs space and privacy just as any other adolescent or adult does. It may also be that they have conflicting and confusing feelings over moral issues. Many young adults now have sexual relations before marriage. Some of them have the privacy to bring people into their bedrooms. If they wish to live together they may set up home together or they may be allowed to have a partner living in the parental home. If the parent does not agree with their sexual behaviour on moral or any other grounds the young adult has the choice to go outside and pursue their activities. They are also at liberty to go to health professionals for contraceptive and sex education and advice. This may not be the case for disabled people. They may be physically dependent on their parents for toileting, dressing and mobility and so it is more difficult for them to assert their needs and it may be more difficult for their parents to let go.

This may be even more difficult for parents of children with mental disability. Parents may find themselves being extremely protective on their children's behalf. In the West, as was mentioned in an earlier chapter, there are no definitive rites of passage for adolescents to become recognized as adults, so it becomes a matter of social judgement dependent on factors such as age, social maturity and IQ. People who have an intellectual impairment may never be able to achieve adult status within our society because they cannot fulfil the criteria. They will always be thought of as a child and protected as such. Unfortunately because of the prevalence of the Western view that children are asexual beings this leads to a denial of the disabled person's sexuality. Obviously there will be individual differences, but overall many of these people will not be educated in sexual matters (particularly those such as eroticism that are learned from alternative sources) and will be restricted in their ability to exercise sexual freedom.

Others, who may not actually be treated as a child may be treated as a perpetual adolescent who is physically, but not emotionally mature, and who is certainly not capable of taking responsibility in sexual matters. Obviously there is an implicit, if not stated, worry that the disabled person will be responsible for bringing another life into the world and one that he or she is unfit to look after properly. There may even be a worry that the disability is hereditary and another impaired person will be born needing a lot of care. These fears cannot be dismissed out of hand but it would seem more useful to acknowledge the person's sexuality and, as is happening more and more today, give them education and knowledge about safe sex and social etiquette (e.g. private not public masturbation) rather than ignoring the issue altogether. This will enable the person to develop in two ways. They will more easily develop a gender identity and role, and will be more socially equipped to view themselves as a sexual being capable of forming a full relationship with another person. The whole issue of contraception is fraught with ethical and legal dilemmas and the reader is referred to the Mencap (see References for address) and Mind (see References for address) organizations for further exploration of the subject.

The opposite side to this coin is that mentally impaired people may be seen by neighbours and others to be a threat to the community and to children in particular. This can be very distressing for the family, although there is little truth in it according to the latest research. This maintains that there is no scientific data that,

the mentally handicapped have no control over their sexuality or have higher sex drives. These individuals sometimes do get into trouble because they have not been taught basic social rules, such as not touching their genitals in public. If they do get into legal trouble, 95 per cent of the time it is for non-violent offences such as 'indecent exposure'. (Reinisch and Beasley, 1991)

Again this may be overcome by a programme of social sex education (and ideally a more general education of the public).

Institutional life may pose problems for disabled people. Even short periods of hospitalization can have stressful effects on the individual because of the loss of privacy and control over their bodily functions. It can lead to a loss of self-identity and the acceptance of a passive role. Sexual intimacy with another person is one way in which identity and self-worth can be affirmed (Savage, 1987) and this may not be possible in short-term institutional care settings and may not be encouraged in long-term establishments. It may not be possible purely because of practical issues, such as lack of transport or child care facilities for the non-hospitalized partner. The needs of people in long-term institutional care may raise issues which their carers and nurses in particular might find challenging, such as whether nurses should physically help disabled people to gain sexual relief? It is recognized by the nursing models that are used, and Roper, Logan and Tierney's model (1985) in particular, that patients are sexual beings and one of the activities of daily living which should be considered is the need to express sexuality. However the dilemma is always there. Whilst the use of a model may show up, as part of the assessment process, just what restrictions there are upon the patient and his or her needs in relation to expressing sexuality, it usually leaves the nurse with the goal of achieving gender attributes, e.g. helping a woman to feel attractive by the use of perfume, cosmetics and appealing bed wear. What it does not do is address the issues involved in achieving sexual, erotic and sensual satisfaction. This can be addressed to a certain extent by use of the PLISTT model (Annon, 1976) which was developed as a tool for sexual health interventions but can be used, if only partially, in the wider sphere of health care.

There are two main factors mentioned earlier that mitigate against people with a disabling condition in relation to sexuality and they may both be present. These are mental and physical difficulties in the achievement of sexual relief and expression. Physical difficulties may be due to paralysis, limitation of movement, absence of limbs, spasticity and weakness. There may be physical attributes, such as scarring or urinary incontinence, which in themselves will not interfere with sexual performance, but may have a profound effect on the person's mental state and which will affect self-concept and sexual behaviour and may even result in sexual dysfunction.

Psychological difficulties may result from one particular aspect of modern society, which is the obsession with the body beautiful. The body in modern mythology has to conform to a set of ideal specifications which do not include physical handicap. This results in disabled people being conditioned into seeing their bodies in a negative light. Sometimes this is done by well-meaning people hoping to protect them from life's knocks, but at other times there can be deliberate cruelty. For example, there may be sarcastic remarks about their perceived incompetence or there may be even more nasty remarks such as telling disabled people that any physically able person who wants to enter a relationship with them does so only out of pity or curiosity. This sort of behaviour can be devastating and result in the need for counselling. Various writers (Nass and Fisher, 1988) have drawn attention to the rights of physically disabled people to draw upon health care resources in order to continue to grow sexually in face of the challenges that they face. They also point out that ablebodiness may be a very temporary affair for anyone . It can be changed in a split second by the 'skid of the motor cycle or car, one invasive virus, one wrong twist of the body while working or playing or by one senseless accident' (*op. cit.*).

It is easy to forget how sensitive all people are in the area of sexuality and how such things as loss of libido or failure to get or maintain an erection may be due to fear and anxiety. This is particularly so in the young or poorly informed disabled person and particularly so when they have been fed a constant diet of goal orientated sex values. Or they may have been given very rigid stereotypes as gender role models which has constantly emphasized the importance of penile-vaginal penetrative intercourse as the only true means of sexual function, but, as anybody who deals with the sexual side of life knows, an erect penis is not the be all and end all of a sexual relationship.

Counselling may help disabled people but it must be done by experienced, sensitive, realistic people. Most disabled people can be helped to achieve a good self-image and a good sex life, but for others it is not always possible. This is because physically disabled people, like ablebodied people represent the whole range of society. It is wrong to stereotype people and categorize them as thinking or acting in a certain way simply because of a disability. People are people, and they have various and different values, opinions and moral attitudes which make it impossible to generalize, particularly in an area as sensitive and personal as sexuality. They may not have a partner and dearly want one, or they may be quite happy without. It has also to be faced that a person may never be able to resume their sex life as it was before an accident or an illness. They may also have to face the fact that their ablebodied partner may not want to assume a different role in the sexual relationship, or that there are aspects of sexuality such as oral-genital sex that they do not want to try. However, enough of this doom and gloom, there are problems and there are solutions. If a person is treated in an individualistic, holistic fashion then there is more often than not a way around any sexual problem, for as has often been pointed out, the most erogenous zone of the body is the mind. Having said that people need to be treated individually it may be useful to mention a few general physical problems and offer suggestions for their resolution. For more help than is within the scope of this book the reader is referred to SPOD (see References for address).

Paralysis and spinal cord injuries give rise to concerns for men about difficulty in achieving an erection and ejaculation and the possibility of reduced spermatogenesis. It is not possible to generalize, but studies have shown that the level of the lesion is of importance in the future ability to achieve and maintain and erection. It seems tthat it is more favourable if the lesion is above T12. There is also some evidence (Savage, 1987) that men can attain an erection from psychogenic stimulation, i.e. cognitive stimulation, but they are usually only of a partial nature. The ability to ejaculate is lost in approximately 90 per cent of men with spinal lesions and when it does occur it is more often of the emission type rather than the expulsive. This is not to say that spinal injured men cannot and do not have an orgasmic type response because such men have been observed to demonstrate the same cardiovascular, pulmonary and muscular changes in the uninvolved part of their bodies as is described by Masters and Johnson as part of the sexual response pattern. Testosterone production seems to continue in much the same vein as before and so a reduction in libido is more often due to factors such as loss of sensation and practical and mental problems such as depression.

Women who have suffered a spinal lesion often develop a significant increase in sensitivity to erotic stimuli in other parts of their bodies, e.g. the breasts, than before and are a capable of orgasmic changes. What they do not tend to have any more is the vaso pelvic congestion and vaginal lubrication changes associated with orgasm. This does not pose too great a problem because it does not prevent penile-vaginal intercourse and a lubricant gel can be used to overcome dryness.

Spasticity and rigidity may result from many different causes such as spinal injury (although not as often as one would think) and cerebral palsy. Cerebral palsy shows itself in a varying fashion from very minor to major manifestations with or without mental retardation. Problems may arise in adolescence mainly due to anxiety about appearance or speech impediments and the anxiety is self-perpetuating in that it can cause reflex spasticity, which in turn will give rise to further anxiety. People with epilepsy may have similar fears in that they are unable to relax in case they have an attack. Counselling may help some cases.

There are other physical disabilities which affect sexual functioning such as multiple sclerosis, muscular dystrophy and poliomyelitis. These tend to give rise to muscle weakness and tiredness, which can lead to loss of libido and an inability to maintain sexual function. Sometimes diabetes or respiratory diseases such as asthma or emphysema have a similar effect. Respiratory troubles may give rise to any number of sexual problems. For example, it may be so difficult to breathe that the thought of breathing rapidly as part of the excitation phase may be extremely frightening and off-putting. Again it is not possible to give general advice that will suit everyone, but people suffering from such problems should visit their general practitioner to discuss their sexual problems specifically and if necessary be referred to a specialist physician for the condition and perhaps to a psychosexual counsellor for the sexual problem. It may be helpful in the meantime if they have a good rest before attempting sexual intercourse and allow their partner to take the active role.

Sometimes people who have had a stroke or a coronary are very scared of being sexually active because they are frightened of having another attack. They will be advised when they can resume by their doctor and there is some evidence to show that it, like any moderate activity is good for them. Some people worry about the rise in blood pressure associated with orgasm. The sufferer will be advised by the doctor to monitor themselves just as they do with any exercise, so that if they develop chest pain or feel distressed they should not resume sexual activity until they have gained their doctor's opinion once more. There may be some residual weakness following a stroke due to damaged nerve pathways and there may be some erectile difficulties in men. There is usually every reason to think that a satisfying sex life is once more possible. Sexual function usually returns fairly quickly after a stroke and if the person can work with his or her partner to find suitable alternative positions and does not feel too hopeless or de-pressed then the difficulties can be overcome.

Arthritis, both osteo and rheumatoid, but perhaps rheumatoid in par-ticular, can present problems for people by limiting their sexual activi-ties. It can be a very painful condition which is characterized by very painful, swollen joints which can make the sufferer lose sexual desire and libido. It is particularly a problem for women and arthritic hip joints may make conventional positions such as the missionary almost impossible. It may be that a rear entry position where the woman lies on her side with her knees drawn up and the man enters from behind may be less of a strain. Or the couple could each lie on their side facing each other. This does not put too much of a strain on either and does not necessitate the woman to have her hips fully abducted. Of course there are other activities that they may wish to try such as oral-genital sex. They may also consider using lots of large, soft pillows to give support without putting pressure on the swollen joints and an electric underblanket will give warmth. Some therapists advise a waterbed if finances permit. (A water bed can be very useful for paralysed people because the ripple effect gives a semblance of physi-cal, response to the thrusting movements.)

Surgery can cause sexual dysfunction for a number of reasons. Some surgery which may be considered to be mutilating, such as mastec-tomy or the creation of an ileostomy or colostomy, can have devastat-ing effects on self-image and self-concept. In the case of ostomies there may be particular problems with fear of leakage and smell which will make the wearer embarrassed and inhibited. There may be a problem of dysfunction due to damage to the pelvic nerves during the resection which can cause post-surgical problems, but the incidence is very small. Most patients in this country have access to aftercare by a qualified stoma nurse who will.give advice on all aspects of care including sexuality.

Interestingly, it need not be totally negative because some people experience a resiting of erogenous zones and there have been reports of the rim of the ostomy becoming quite sensitive to touch in an erotic way.

Following a mastectomy, a woman may become quite depressed and feel insecure. This may be in part due to the fear of the cancer that necessitated the removal of the breast, but obviously a change in body image does not help. Some surgeons may offer to place an implant at the time of surgery and this will, in part, mitigate the problem. Other women may be offered breast reconstruction at later date or may simply choose to wear an insert in a specially designed bra. Whatever they choose, for most women there is always a need for extra reassurance after a mastectomy and a warm loving partner will help in the healing process. This may also be the case following a hysterectomy even though there may be no outward signs. Many women do not understand the anatomy of their bodies and fear the resumption of sexual intercourse. Indeed some women do not know that they will have a vagina just as before. Some women mourn their ability to bear children and some may fear that their partner's penis is going to undo the stitches in some way. All these fears can be allayed to a greater or lesser degree by education and/or counselling. There is no evidence to suggest that women cannot have a full sex life after a hysterectomy and this is the case for most types of vaginal surgery, such as colporrhaphy, except where there has been artificial narrowing of the introitus and the presence of scar tissue causes subsequent pain on intercourse (dyspareunia).

One of the problems with being disabled may be the need to take drugs, and some drugs have a negative effect on sexual functioning. They are many and varied and it is not possible to give a list of drugs and their effects. If a person has a problem and has been prescribed a drug by his or her medical practitioner, the doctor should be asked for information about the drug and in particular any possible side-effects on sexual activity. Otherwise the individual may not connect the dysfunction with the drug and may simply lose interest in sex and give up. Having said this there are certain groups of drugs that it is possible to generalize about, such as sedatives. In small doses sedatives, hypnotics and tranquillisers, for example diazepam, may cause relaxation and release inhibitions or free the individual from anxiety. In large doses they will depress the libido and functioning. Some adrenergic blocking drugs prescribed for hypertension, may cause ejaculatory problems although they may not interfere with desire or erectile ability in men. It may be possible that anticonvulsants result in a loss in libido in epileptic men but a causal relationship has not been proven. Other drugs such as digoxin have an effect on the endocrine glands and may result in reduced sexual activity. There are leisure drugs both legal and illegal such as alcohol, marijuana, ecstasy and cocaine that will have an effect on sexual functioning but it is not proposed to detail them here except to say that alcohol is notorious for increasing desire and decreasing performance. It is also related to problems in spermatogenesis and teratogenesis which gives rise to the birth of a congenitally damaged infant suffering from the fetal alcohol syndrome.

A complication of disability may be the impairment of the ability to procreate, i.e. a reduction in fertility. This is not the case for everyone and again it is worth reiterating that people are individuals and there is a wide spectrum of fertility in any given population. Normally, in order to achieve a satisfactory pregnancy certain conditions have to be satisfied. They are as follows:

- the production of a mature ovum which is released into the fallopian tubes;
- the production of sufficient, motile, spermatazoa which are deposited in the vagina around the time of ovulation;
- fertilization of the ovum in the Fallopian tubes and healthy ciliated tubal epithelium to waft the morula towards the uterus;
- a healthy uterus with a thick endometrium to provide a nourishing environment for the embryo/fetus;
- hormonal balance.

It can be seen by examining each condition that there may be factors that interfere with the process. For example, if there is hormonal imbalance the process may simply not begin or it may not be completed. Either the male or the female will not produce mature ova or spermatazoa, or there will be a tendency to miscarry. There is nothing here that is peculiar to physically disabled people but certain drugs may inhibit ovulation or spermatogenesis. (They may be dangerous to a developing fetus and so it is always necessary to have preconceptional counselling before embarking on a pregnancy.) Some mentally disabling conditions such as Down's and Klinefelter's syndromes are associated with hormonal anomalies and subsequent sterility. Others, particularly those which have resulted from birth trauma, are not associated with either sterility or hereditary problems.

Ovulation is not usually affected by physical disabilities including spinal injuries providing, of course, the ovaries, Fallopian tubes or uterus have not been damaged. After the initial lesion menstruation usually returns with a few months and pregnancy and vaginal delivery are possible as before. (There may be a tendency to urinary tract infections in pregnancy but that is all.) Spermatogenesis is more problematic. Following a spinal injury there is very often a reduction in spermatogenesis and the sperm produced may have a reduced motility. This could be due in part to the higher temperature of the testes because of sitting in a wheelchair. Ejaculation and deposition of the spermatazoa in the vagina may also be a problem. This may not be insuperable because it may be possible to produce ejaculation by electrical stimulation of the pelvic nerves through the rectum. The sperm thus collected can be used to inseminate the partner either by straightforward deposition in the vagina or even by IVF (in-vitro fertilisation). Even if there is a low sperm count the sperm from several ejaculates can be collected, frozen and pooled together for later use. Fertility treatment is making great strides and there are many documented cases of spinal cord injured men fathering children. Likewise disabled women should not think of themselves as not being able to have children. There may be difficulties but human nature being what it is there is always a way round things, particularly if one has enough support.

PART THREE

The Raison D'Etre

CHAPTER SEVEN

Pregnant and Sexually Active

Expectant, round and heavy with child,
Silently deep and brimming with life
Magnificent strong and proudly wild
Nearer to nature than culture's wife.
I Walton. Proudly Awaiting

To do or not to do! That seems to be the question (with apologies to Shakespeare) when it comes to considering sexual intercourse and pregnancy. It is not so long ago that the answer was simple, 'don't'. Why this answer was given, was however, very complicated and not at all related to fact or research, but was an amalgamation of old wives tales and personal moral stances based on very dubious cultural hand-me-downs. So, how is a professional now to respond to the question of whether and when a woman should have or should not have sex in pregnancy? With commonsense, compassion and a good background knowledge, one hopes. It may be useful at this point to examine the stages of pregnancy, concentrating on the physical factors, particularly the common worries and problems that may arise.

Pregnancy is often considered in three parts or trimesters. In fact, there is no real distinction between these as stages but the demarcation is useful in order to consider particular worries and problems in relation to sexuality. Before going into detail it must be emphasized that there is no 'norm' of sexual behaviour particularly when thinking about pregnancy. The activities of couples in this area vary from none at all to a vastly increased level.

In the first few weeks after conception sexual activity for many people goes on as before, simply because they do not know the woman is pregnant. After a few weeks when the pregnancy is beginning to make itself obvious either by breast tingling and feelings of water

75

retention or by nausea and vomiting, women may react in one of two ways. They may feel liberated and extremely libidinous, or they may find that being pregnant has reduced their sexual desires. The pelvic congestion associated with pregnancy may have the effect of increasing desire and for some women it enables them to experience orgasm for the first time. For others there is a fear of harming the fetus and an associated avoidance of orgasm. The breasts of a nulliparous woman undergo an increase of approximately 25 per cent in the plateau period of sexual activity (Masters and Johnson, 1966), and by the end of the first trimester of pregnancy have undergone a similar increase in size. So when there is the added dimensions of sexual activity and pregnancy the resultant 50 per cent increase does cause some women to complain of discomfort. Backache is a significant factor in many women's pregnancies and it can occur after coitus, but although not usually of any great significance, it can be upsetting and worrying. Some women also complain of a slight ache after intercourse in the midline over the pubic area. This could be due to one or both of two factors, either as an orgasmic response in the uterus itself or tension on the round ligaments of the uterus as the uterus takes on a more upright and rounded shape.

Early pregnancy is a time when women very often report that they feel very tired and so for working women their desire may decrease because of this lethargy. It may be that some women lose interest in sex because they associate it with a desire for pregnancy. Now this has been achieved they do not feel the need to continue with the activity. Quite simply they may not love their partner or they may dislike sexual intercourse for any of a number of reasons. If it is because of a long-standing sexual problem such as pain or psychological reasons then the problem will not be resolved by pregnancy but simply postponed for a while. If the partner is not a skilful lover and the woman is constantly disappointed then pregnancy may be used as an excuse to reduce the chance of discontentment. Or it may be simply that the woman is worried and frightened. This is particularly so if there is a history of infertility or miscarriage. She or her partner may worry that they will harm the fetus in some way or other. Although research into the effect of sexual intercourse has been limited there is no evidence (Behrman, Kistner and Patton, 1988) to suggest that it is a significant factor in miscarriage.

Male partners may also worry that they may do some harm to the fetus, and a small minority have the opposite worry, that the fetus will damage them. Some men seem to experience the symptoms of pregnancy with their partner (couvade) and if they are feeling nauseous and head achey they too will have a reduction in libidinous feelings. If a man worries that he may be hurting his partner or damaging his unborn baby then it may be quite difficult for him to gain and maintain an erection. This, in itself, will be troubling but if the pair keep a sense of proportion it will not progress to a habit and become a psycho-sexual problem. It is easier to keep it in perspective if one is well informed. So it behoves the professionals, and particularly the mid-wife, to give information about sex in pregnancy in as factual and objective a way as all other advice in pregnancy is given.

It may be that the man is very sympathetic and will be very supportive to his partner to the extent of curtailing his sexual drive, even when there is no need to do so. It may be that he is very sensitive and anxious about the safety of the pregnancy and sees his role as the protector and guardian of his family, which causes him to limit him-self. This is no problem if his partner understands and concurs with his decision, but many women are lacking in assurance in pregnancy and need a lot of convincing that they are desirable so this is no time for abstinence. Although some religions have a number of prohibi-tions about sexual intercourse during menstruation and after childbirth few are very prescriptive about sex in pregnancy. However, indi-vidual couples may decide for themselves that their religious or cul-tural background prevents them from having sex during this time. Again it must be emphasized that if they are both happy with the situation then there is no problem. Other unhappy inhibiting factors for a man may be that he does not believe he is the father of the unborn baby and may feel cheated and betrayed. This, of course, may be true or may not be, but the feelings the man experiences will be enough to put him off sex. Another way of feeling deceived is when the woman has stopped using contraceptives without the man's knowledge, lead-ing to a wanted pregnancy on her part but a time of turmoil for her partner. Until he resolves his feelings he may lose desire for her. This may be particularly the case with young teenagers who were experi-menting with sex rather than maturely deciding to bring another life into the world.

Being pregnant is not all sexually negative and many couples find that it is the greatest turn-on ever. The woman feels fulfilled and magnificent and the man feels proud and protective. The fear of pregnancy has gone, so there is no need to use contraceptives which may have been irksome. Pelvic congestion and an increase in oestrogen and progesterone result in an increased lubrication of the vagina and the woman, as was said earlier, may experience a heightened response and for some it may be the first time that they have experienced orgasm.

As pregnancy progresses it brings with it similarly diverse reactions as those described for the first trimester. In the second trimester the woman's shape is noticeably changing and this will bring either positive or negative reactions, or a mixture of both to the fore. How the couple react to the changes depends very much on their attitudes to body shape in general and to the pregnancy. It is not really possible to be definitive but there are a few common reactions. Some women are really proud of their 'bump' and take the first opportunity they can to wear maternity clothes that announce their condition. Others feel that they have become fat and continue to play down the development for as long as possible. Likewise with men, some adore the look of pregnant woman and find them extremely attractive, whilst others simply do not. It is all a matter of individual taste, socialization and religious and cultural upbringing. What is unfortunate is when there is a mixture of attitudes within the partnership which causes unhappiness for one or other of the partners.

In the main, the second trimester is one of heightened sexual awareness and eroticism. For most women the minor disorders of pregnancy have ceased, they no longer feel quite so tired and they may have finished working The fear of miscarriage which is strongest in the early weeks has passed and they are not yet so big that they find lying down a problem. The labia majora and minora although generally vaso congested are not usually oedematous and uncomfortable. There is an almost constant discharge, the leucorrhoea of pregnancy, that ensures ease of penetration. (This discharge is clear to whitish in colour, does not irritate and is not offensive in smell.) There is however no secretion from the cervix, the cervical os is closed by a thick mucous plug, the operculum, which is formed under the influence of progesterone, and which effectively seals off the uterine cavity from the outside world and acts as a protection against infection. The venous congestion of pregnancy results in a heightened manifestation of all aspects of the sexual act so that the area becomes congested, the orgasm is heightened and the vaginal lumen becomes smaller thus gripping the penis tighter. There is also a tendency for the uterus to contract but these contractions do not seem to be harmful. On the contrary they are of the Braxton-Hicks type and probably perfuse the uterus with blood.

There is a sharp decrease in sexual activity in the third trimester (Kenny, 1976). This is due to many factors but in the main is associated with the discomforts of late pregnancy. These include sleeplessness and tiredness, backache, oedema of the vulva, haemorrhoids and frequency of micturition. There may also be medical conditions in some women that mitigate against increased sexual activity. These include diabetes mellitus with its accompanying and irritating monilial infections, hypertension and oedema, and urinary problems. Some women report an overall lack of interest in sex, and an overwhelming preoccupation with the unborn baby and the prospect of the delivery. This is particularly so as the estimated date of confinement draws near or is passed. There is also the worry that intercourse will bring on a premature labour or injure the fetus in some way. It can also be very frightening if there is spotting of blood after intercourse, which is quite likely in late pregnancy due to the friability of the extremely engorged cervical mucosa.

The man may also be quite worried about causing damage to the baby and find that his desire is reduced because of it. Some couples have reported (Close, 1984) that the man becomes sexually inhibited because they feel a 'third' person is present. Some men find the physical changes of late pregnancy offputting and there is a reduction in their libido, or they may find alternative outlets for sexual expression. This may be simply an increase in masturbation, but some men, particularly where there are existing problems with the relationship, will opt for sexual intercourse outside the partnership.

Most of the fears and worries that preoccupy couples when the woman is pregnant fall into two camps. They are: the fear of miscarriage, premature labour and damage to the baby; and the worry about infections and conditions in the pregnancy. The threat of miscarriage is a common and recurring worry for many, particularly if it has happened to them before. In general miscarriage occurs because there is an abnormality in the developing ovum or the reproductive organs, a depletion in the production of the necessary hormones such as progesterone or, rarely, an accident. There is no evidence to suggest that sexual intercourse in the absence of any of the predisposing factors will cause miscarriage. Obviously women who have a history of early miscarriage, vaginal spotting, or pain would be advised to consult their general practitioner, but for the majority of women there is no need to worry. The same advice can be given with regard to premature labour. The mechanism of onset of labour is imperfectly understood but there are several factors that must come together. The placenta produces a hormone throughout pregnancy, progesterone, which maintains the pregnancy. A hormone oxytocin is produced by the posterior pituitary gland which opposes progesterone and causes smooth muscle to contract. The placenta produces an enzyme, oxytocinase, which breaks down oxytocin and so neutralizes its action. In late pregnancy as the placenta starts to decline, the balance of these hormones changes and the uterus becomes irritable, i.e. it can be made to contract quite easily. In addition there is localized production of prostaglandins at the cervix which enhances the effect of oxytocin. These factors in conjunction with the increased size of the uterus comprise a situation favourable for the onset of labour. It can be seen that it is unlikely that sexual intercourse will cause onset of a labour where the factors were not in place anyway. At the end of pregnancy semen which contains prostaglandins may bathe the cervix and facilitate the action of the oxytocin from the pituitary gland. The uterus may be induced to contract during orgasm and again this may facilitate the onset of labour, but is not enough in itself if the other factors are not present. So it can be said that sex in late pregnancy is unlikely to start premature labour but may be a fun way to start labour at term or beyond. It is highly unlikely that the fetus will be endangered by such activity, although in a compromised pregnancy, uterine contractions in themselves may cause a deceleration in the fetal heart rate. Also it should be avoided if there is bleeding or ruptured membranes.

One of the problems associated with fear for the baby is the lack of knowledge about practices in pregnancy. It is not enough (although it is often said) for professionals to tell the couple to be careful. What is careful? Most people do not know, so they make up their own rules as they go along. There are only two practices that should not be undertaken. One of these is blowing air into the vagina. As was said in an earlier chapter, cunnilingus in itself is not harmful if it is restricted to oral stimulation of the clitoris and external genitalia. It is unlikely to cause damage because the operculum will prevent air entering the uterus. However the danger is that what is normal for one couple may be extremely abnormal for another, so it must be stressed that forceful blowing of air into the vagina may be highly dangerous. The other practice that should not be done is the insertion of foreign bodies into the vagina particularly in a forceful manner. Apart from the physical danger of piercing the vaginal walls or damaging the cervical os there is a risk of altering the pH balance of the vaginal walls and cause infection. Fellatio is not dangerous because even though semen contains prostaglandins it is not a problem if swallowed due to the action of the stomach acid.

Some positions in pregnancy are uncomfortable rather than dangerous, although the missionary position can be problematic. As the pregnancy progresses the enlarged uterus may press on the inferior vena cava when the woman lies on her back. It impedes venous return and can result in a drop in the blood pressure and a fainting attack. This will be compounded if the woman is lying on her back with the weight of her partner on top as well. It is probably better as pregnancy advances to make use of positions where the woman is on top, i.e. either sitting on his knee or straddling him whilst he lies on his back. The distinct advantage of 'woman on top' positions is that the woman can also control the depth of penetration. It is less likely that she will experience discomfort during coitus. Another method may be a rear entry position with the woman either kneeling or lying in the spoon position.

It is worth remembering here that sexual intercourse does not necessarily mean that one must indulge in penetrative sex. For couples who do not choose to carry on with penile-vaginal intercourse or who have been advised against it for some reason there are always alternatives. These can include masturbation, both self and mutual stimulation, oral sex, deep massage or simply kissing and cuddling. There is no right way and there is nothing wrong with experimentation unless one of the couple is not happy with the proposed practices.

The fears about infection are very often unfounded because for the most part they are based on old wives tales rather than fact. As was said earlier, the normal leucorrhoea of pregnancy is whitish to clear in colour, odourless and non-irritant. So any woman who has a discharge which is different from this, i.e. is profuse, coloured (it can be greenish, brownish or yellowish), or causes itching or inflammation, must be seen by a doctor. The most common deviation from normal is a monilial infection (candida albicans or thrush). This occurs when the ph of the vagina becomes more alkaline or when the tissues are high in glycogen such as is the case in diabetes or when a course of antibiotics kills off the commensal organisms of the vagina. It is characterized by a white cheesy type of discharge which is highly irritating. Women report that the itching can be so intense that they scratch themselves till it bleeds. The infection can make a woman lose sleep and become quite run down. However, it is easily treatable. One form of prevention is to wear cotton underwear and avoid nylon tights because the organism thrives in warm, moist places. Men are not, in general, prone to thrush but it can be harboured under the foreskin, so it is as well if the woman has it for the man to be treated as well.

Other infections which may be contracted in pregnancy are the sexually transmitted diseases (STDs) of which the most common are trichomonas vaginalis, gonorrhoea, syphilis, chlamydia, non specific urethritis, herpes, and of course, the latest scourge of mankind, AIDS and the HIV infection. The problem with any discussion about sexually transmitted diseases is that they are fenced around with cultural and social taboos. So finding out that one's partner is infected with gonorrhoea, for instance, is not thought of in a similar light to finding out that he or she has a staphylococcal infection, even though the causative organisms are very similar. In general, because they are sexually transmitted, the non-infected partner within a relationship may become infected because the other partner has been infected from another source. This can obviously put a considerable strain on the relationship which is serious at any time, but is heightened when the woman is pregnant. In general, women are more likely to contract a STD following an act of intercourse than men are.

This makes a pregnant woman within a relationship particularly at risk because she may not be expecting her partner to use a condom. Having said this, it is necessary to point out the assumption, which will not be correct for a number of women, that they are actually in a relationship and that they or their partner are monogamous. Any high risk behaviour, such as unprotected vaginal or anal sexual intercourse or indeed any activity such as oral genital sex, which exposes a man or woman to another's bodily secretions may be considered high risk. The only exception is when the two are in an exclusive monogamous relationship and both are definitely not infected.

Trichomonas Vaginalis is caused by a protozoa parasite which usually causes a greenish yellow, highly irritant, profuse, purulent discharge with itching (pruritis) and inflammation, but occasionally there may be no symptoms at all. It may also cause a urethritis, particularly in the man. It is diagnosed by examining a swab under the microscope for the flagellated protozoa. Another common feature is painful intercourse (dyspareunia) for both the man and the woman. It is sexually transmitted and so the both partners need to be treated by the doctor. The drug of choice at this moment in time is metronidazole (flagyl) but this may be teratogenic (cause fetal abnormalities) and so is contraindicated in pregnancy (particularly in the first trimester) and lactation, so clotrimazole pessaries and cream may be prescribed instead.

Gonorrhoea is a bacterial infection caused by the neisseria gonococcal which is a gram negative organism. It results in a purulent green discharge from the penis or the vagina after an incubation period which can vary from one day to three weeks. The treatment is by large doses of ampicillin with probenecid. If untreated it can spread right up the reproductive tract causing salpingitis and eventually pelvic inflammatory disease. If contracted in early pregnancy it can result in a miscarriage but after the first trimester it does not tend to ascend because of the effectiveness of the operculum as a barrier. However when the fetus passes through the vagina at delivery it is in danger of being contaminated and of contracting a gonococcal ophthalmia. This can cause a pustular discharge from the eyes within hours of birth and which if not treated with antibiotics will rapidly cause blindness in the baby.

Syphilis is caused by the spirochaete, Treponema Pallidum, which enters the blood stream via a crack in the mucosa. It is most often a sexually transmitted disease but can be acquired in other ways, for example, by midwives who handle the placenta of an infected mother without protection. There are four stages in the course of the disease. The primary stage is characterized by the appearance of a small hard sore or chancre between nine and 90 days after infection, which may be present upon the penis or in the vagina or on the cervix. It is circular with a raised rim and a depression in the centre. During this stage the disease is extremely infectious. The chancre may heal up in about six weeks but this does not mean that the person is cured, quite the contrary in fact. The secondary stage begins a few weeks later and is characterized by a feeling of being unwell and generally under the weather with flu-like symptoms, sore throat and aches and pains. There may be a rash which occurs after the chancre has healed and is brownish-red in colour and distributed over the body and chest and upper arms in particular. Contact with this rash can result in infection. Flat large warts, condylomata, may appear on the vulva. (Vulval warts are not necessarily syphilitic in origin, they are more commonly caused by the papilloma virus and are treated by cryosurgery in pregnancy. The woman is followed up by annual cervical smears as the papilloma virus has been associated with cervical carcinoma.) Syphilitic warts look like a flat grey type of mushroom and can smell quite offensive. If the condition is untreated it appears to go into remission and a latency stage occurs which can last for years. During this time the disease is not contagious and the spirochaetes although still infecting the body seem to have little effect. The exception to this rule is that of a pregnant woman, who will pass the infection across the placenta to the fetus which will be born with congenital syphilis. In the fourth and final stage there is very serious damage to the individual where ulcer type lesions, the gummata, can be present anywhere in the body and the individual may be paralysed or have locomotor ataxia with or without a severe psychiatric disorder (general paralysis of the insane - GPI). As the treponema pass through the placenta it infects it and reduces its efficiency which, in itself, is detrimental to the health of the fetus. In addition, the fetus becomes infected and if born alive has characteristic problems. These include damage to the nose and to the mucous membranes of the mouth resulting in a depression at the bridge of the nose (saddle nose) and constant snuffles. Cracks at the side of the mouth can be present, as can be damage to the tooth buds resulting in deformed (Hutchinson's) teeth. There may be a pemphigus type rash and damage to the liver and the spleen. Without treatment the baby will continue to deteriorate, but with penicillin the damage can be halted but not reversed. Syphilis can be treated with large doses of penicillin quite successfully whenever it is diagnosed. It is screened for in all pregnant women in the British Isles by the use of VDRL slide tests (Venereal Disease Research Laboratory) or the RPR (Rapid Plasma Reagin) and the TPHA (Treponema Pallidum Haemaglutination) test. It is confirmed by the use of the FTA (Fluorescent Treponema Antibody test. Contact tracing is done and the contacts of the infected person are offered blood tests and treatment if necessary (Holmes *et al*, 1990).

Chlamydia trachomatis is a bacterial infection that is parasitic, i.e. it lives within a host cell. It is a major factor in the infection of the reproductive organs of both sexes and is a factor in the development of pelvic inflammatory disease. It may be symptomless for a long time even though it causes scarring and damage, particularly to the Fallopian tubes. Even when there are symptoms they may be overlooked because the resultant issue may be simply a watery, thin discharge. It is thought to be responsible for a substantial proportion of the non-specific urethritis in men. It can also cause pneumonia or an eye infection in the fetus as it passes through the birth canal and the resultant trachoma (eye infection) can lead to permanent blindness. It can be screened for by the Abbot test pack which gives result from a cervical smear in approximately 30 minutes with a high rate of effectiveness. Once diagnosed it can be treated quite successfully with tetracyclines. This is contraindicated in pregnancy so erythromycin is usually administered instead.

Herpes is another condition that may be sexually transmitted. It is caused by the herpes simplex virus HSV-2, which is related to the virus that causes cold sores herpes simplex HSV-1, and which causes genital sores. When a person first contracts genital herpes they have what is termed the primary eruption which is probably the most painful phase of the condition. It is characterized by pain on micturition, itching and a vaginal or cervical discharge. They are likely to feel unwell with headaches, stiff neck and sensitivity to light. They also have blister type sores on the penis or cervix, in the vagina and round the anus and the urethra. The fluid from the blisters is very infectious and anyone who comes into contact with them is at risk. The condition then goes into remission and there can be long periods without an outbreak but the virus is still within the cells. On average people will have about five episodes each year in the first two years. Recurrent infections do not tend to be as severe as the primary episode. The virus can be transmitted to the fetus in pregnancy but usually only when the mother is suffering from a primary episode, recurrent episodes do not seem to be as infectious in pregnancy to the fetus. There does seem to be a higher than average risk of miscarrying or premature delivery due to the presence of a primary outbreak, but not with recurrent episodes. It used to be thought that any woman with a history of genital herpes should have a caesarian section to prevent the baby being infected in the journey through the birth canal but the current thinking is that it is only necessary if the mother has an active breakout at term. An infected baby is at risk of developing viral encephalitis which can be fatal. The diagnosis is by physical examination followed by isolation of the virus from the sores. Routine screening in pregnancy is not thought to be a useful exercise and so is not usually undertaken (Kelly, 1988). Diagnosis is usually arrived at from the clinical history and evidence of signs and symptoms. Treatment which is not always effective is by acyclovir which may be given at around 32 weeks of gestation to enable the attack to have cleared up by the time delivery is due.

The final sexually transmitted disease which will be discussed in this book is acquired immunodeficiency syndrome (AIDS) which is thought to be caused by most of the experts by the human immunodeficiency virus (HIV) even though there is a small number of eminent scientists who dispute this as the causative agent. More time is devoted to this condition in Chapter 12.

Before completing the discussion of sex in pregnancy it is worth considering the women who are not pregnant because of a loving (however brief) encounter and those who may be pregnant but are not happy about it. Women may be pregnant as a result of sexual abuse which can be rape, within or without marriage or partnership, or it can be an incestuous relationship within the family. The woman (or for that matter the man) may be an adult survivor of child sexual abuse and pregnancy has been found to be a major trigger for flashbacks (Kitzinger, 1992; Simkin, 1992). Obviously if these factors are involved there may at the very least be ambiguous feelings towards sexual intercourse because the site of the abuse and its musculature is involved in the sexual act. The feelings and fears which will be in evidence may need the help of an experienced counsellor. Many women are the victims of violent men and they may actively strive to maintain a passive state (Hiberman, 1990) because they think that they can control the violence by being good, quiet and compliant. As abusive men can be set off by something as simple as their wife breaking an egg (Shainess, 1984) and pregnancy seems to be a particular trigger (Bewley and Gibbs, 1991) it is no wonder that such women may be quite frightened during sexual intercourse and will not be in a position to refuse unwanted activities nor will they be able to express their own needs. These issues will be considered further in Chapter 10.

CHAPTER EIGHT

Labour, A Sexual Act

And a great portent appeared in the heaven, a woman clothed with the sun, with the moon under her feet, and on her head a crown of twelve stars; she was with child and she cried out in pangs of birth, in anguish for delivery.
Revelation, Ch.12, v.1

Is childbirth sexual and erotic? How could it be? Surely it is about pain and hard work? Of course this cannot be denied, but all the same there is another dimension to it, that of sexuality as expressed through the body. Having the baby is the end point of a process that more often than not began privately enough between two people. They made love, the woman conceived, and for her, and usually for him, began a process that is life changing. During the pregnancy sexuality was expressed in a different and sometimes more intense way than before and then the time of fulfilment arrives. How can it not be sexual and erotic in its own way? The physiological reactions are very similar, the process is genital focused and it is a time of intense emotional responses and involvement. It is strange that this is not recognized, if only by the couple themselves. Perhaps it is, but is not acknowledged and is repressed in both the participants and the attendants. This is not as strange as one would think because attitudes to sexuality are cultivated over a lifespan and one takes on board all manner of cultural and social messages and taboos until they are firmly internalized and become part of oneself. An examination of the process of labour and childbirth is helpful in looking at the way sexuality at this time is, is not and could be expressed.

For many women labour begins many hours before they summon a midwife or go into the maternity unit. It usually begins with a dull period type backache that gradually becomes more intense and develops into contractions that are then felt in the lower abdomen. For others it starts with irregular contractions which are felt as pains in the lower abdomen and which gradually become regular. In some women the contractions may start and then stop for a while and then start again. All that can really be said about the beginning of labour is that each woman is different and each labour is different but there are shared similarities. One of the most frequently shared similarities is a sense of excitement and anticipation. This feeling may be shared with her partner and they both become very exhilarated. When a young couple who care about each other are in a state of excitement and shared animation they are in a state of arousal. This does not mean that they are about to have intercourse, but they might, and perhaps in this case they should. However it is unlikely they will do so unless all is well, they are at home and have the confidence to know that all is well and no harm will be done. The assumption being made here of course is that sexuality and the sexual act is expressed as coitus.

During the first stage of labour the woman may need to be reassured that the labour is progressing well and that she is coping well and is in control of the process. In this she will be helped by a confident partner who is empowered by her attendants to give her all the physical and emotional support possible. One of the important aspects of care in labour is the attempt to relieve pain. Pain is a vicious circle whereby the woman who is in pain can become emotionally and physically distressed with a resultant physiological change which causes more painful contractions, a longer labour and a reduced tolerance (or lowered pain threshold) to pain itself. If the woman is given as much help as possible to keep her tolerance to pain under control and helped to stimulate the brain to release its own natural painkillers (endorphins) then the labour becomes easier. There are two main ways to do this, either by pharmacological methods such as administration of drugs or by non pharmacological methods which stimulate the gate response to pain (Melzack and Wall, 1965).

One of the objectives of the non-pharmacological process is to induce a sense of well-being and confidence and a reduction in stress and tension. This is done by having present people in whom the woman has confidence, and by the use of soothing practices such as relaxation techniques, warm baths, aromatherapy, back rubbing and transcutaneous electrical nerve stimulation (TENS). The ancient remedy of back rubbing is well documented in midwifery textbooks and lectures for student midwives. However, it is described very clinically as a procedure that the partner needs to perform in a certain manner. The coverage given to it is very superficial and runs along the lines of describing how to perform circular massage to the lower back in the latter part of the first stage. Some writers (Flint, 1986; Kitzinger, 1983) have drawn attention to the need for sensitivity in midwifery care and a greater awareness of the need for a cherishing approach to women in labour.

This being so, the partner should not be merely shown how to rub the back with the heel of the hand during a contraction. For there is a danger of back rubbing being seen as a clinical procedure in the same way as being shown how to apply pressure to a wound. This is particularly so if the couple are not given any privacy. Caroline Flint (1986) notes that she has never seen a labour ward that is capable of being locked from the inside and that is also the experience of this author. Even when people knock on labour ward doors as they increasingly tend to do these days, it is not usually a request for admission which can be granted or refused by the occupants, rather it is a warning of intention to enter. Without privacy the couple will not have the freedom to become more intimate and quietly communicative. The atmosphere is not conducive to deep relaxation, particularly in a very busy delivery suite. The midwives are not unaware of this and do try to minimize the distraction but, particularly in the daytime, they can be fighting a losing battle.

Rather than being shown how to rub the lower back it may be better if the couple were given the authority to lock the door, given comfortable surroundings and encouraged to hug, kiss and caress each other. This would have an extremely beneficial effect on the woman in labour. Not only would her anxiety levels be reduced and with it the need for analgesia but the contractions would become more effective. It is well-known that animals in labour seem to be able to choose the time (usually the night) and the place of their delivery in order to gain privacy and that labour may cease if they are disturbed. Although it has been documented (Newton, Peeler and Newton, 1968) for many years that disturbance in labour may lessen uterine contractions in humans very little thought (or further research) is given to it in modern obstetrics. This means that women are at risk of iatrogenically produced diminishment of contractions with its accompanying and inevitable sequelae of intervention.

During the earlier part of the first stage the couple could lie on the bed and perhaps have a sleep together. This does not happen, instead the woman lies on the bed and unless the unit is very enlightened the man has the choice of a chair, which can vary from a very comfortable armchair to a hard plastic stacking one, or if he is lucky, a bean bag. Even where there are beds in the labour room large enough to accommodate both of them, the tendency is for the woman to occupy it alone. There are many arguments for and against having a baby at home but the luxury of being in one's own bed and bedroom, having privacy and its effect on the contractions is a very powerful one in favour. Community midwives have long known that far less pethidine is needed at a home confinement. More than back rubbing would be beneficial and can be given at home. Long stroking movements along the thighs, legs and ankles can be very soothing. As labour progress many women complain of pains down their inner thighs and over the symphysis pubis. These could be alleviated to some extent by their partner stroking the inside of the thigh and over the mons veneris. This would be seen by some couples (and their attendants) as so overtly sexual that they would be totally inhibited without privacy. This is sad because it would be more beneficial in so many ways to both the woman and her unborn baby. It may prove to be an alternative and effective method of pain relief.

Massage is used all over the world to ease the pain of labour. This varies with the culture but it can be a light effleurage, a deep massage, or shiatsu and acupressure, and it can be with or without the aid of oil. Not only is massage of the back and shoulders good but long light stroking over the abdomen and down into the perineal area gives a good feeling of pain relief and well-being. There are many different types of oils, depending on local availability and tradition, but some of the most commonly used are coconut, olive, grapeseed, jojoba or sweet almond. Aromatherapy is being revived in this country and the preceding oils are used as carriers for essential oils which are extracts of plants, usually flowers, which are used therapeutically often in conjunction with massage. Oils (particularly rose and geranium in sweet almond oil) can be used on the back through labour but only once or twice on the abdomen in labour (Worwood, 1992). The oils that are recommended (*op. cit.*) are rose, neroli, lavender, nutmeg, clary sage (not sage) and geranium. Oiling of the perineum is thought to help the perineum to stretch and reduce the incidence of trauma, but the research to date is not conclusive (Avery and Burket, 1986; Mynaugh, 1991). It is, however, (according to anecdotal reports) very relaxing particularly if it is performed by the partner. Again this is a procedure that is so sensual that privacy is essential. Some midwives will massage the perineum with olive oil as the head is crowning in an effort to facilitate stretching and reduce tearing. This procedure is relatively uncommon in this country but is fairly frequent in other parts of the world (Dunham *et al*, 1991). Stimulation of the nipples is another practice that has a place in labour too. It causes a rush of oxytocin from the posterior pituitary gland which will cause the uterus to contract more effectively. It could be performed by the partner as part of the process of labour (Dunham *et al*, 1991), but more often when it is done it is by the midwife to hasten the third stage or cause the uterus to contract. This is to prevent haemorrhage when there is no syntocinon drip in situ or for some reason the midwife is reluctant or unable to use syntometrine or ergometrine as part of the management of the third stage of labour.

As the first stage of labour progresses it becomes physiologically similar to the sexual arousal process in many ways. The woman's blood pressure and her pulse rate may rise slightly. Contractions of labour start to be felt and gradually become more frequent and more intense until they are lasting approximately 60 seconds with the period of relaxation between them reducing until they are two minutes or so apart. There is a feeling of mounting anticipation within the room and for most women it is a time to withdraw into herself. Outside events become no more than an unwelcome distraction and there is a different time span to events. No longer is time a measure of day and night. It becomes labour time, measured by the chronology of labour. It is the woman's body that is dictating the time span, or it should be. As the tension and the intensity of the contractions mounts, some women feel happier if they are immersed in water. This has a soothing, calming and pain relieving effect, particularly when used in a room with subdued lighting and soft music. Most women will use the warm water bath only during the first stage and will want to get out of the bath for the actual delivery. Some may want to stay in the water and deliver there and so if the woman so wishes (unless there are any contraindications) she can do so. Although the safety of water birth delivery has been a controversial topic in the midwifery press the latest information is saying that it is quite a safe procedure for most women (Ingrey, 1993). This being so it can be a source of great comfort to most women and the father may in some cases be able to join his partner in the water if they both so wish.

Some of the procedures that are performed in labour involve the exposure of the woman's genitalia and penetrative vaginal examination by hand or speculum. Many women find these very disturbing and difficult to cope with. There are issues not only of physical pain associated with the procedure but also more subtle psychological factors involving powerlessness and vulnerability. This is particularly so for women who have been sexually abused at some time in the past (Kitzinger, 1992; Grant, 1992; Draucker, 1992). Unfortunately this does not seem to be widely understood by the care givers and vaginal examinations are undertaken in a very ritualistic manner and very often without a clear rationale. They are more often than not performed as part of active management of labour with the frequency determined in an arbitrary and unthinking manner as part of a routine protocol. They could be better and more sensitively performed and less frequently used (Bergstrom *et al*, 1992). There is little if anything in midwifery or obstetric textbooks to bring the professional's attention to the psychological effects of what can be physically little different from abuse. Nor does it seem to be understood that there is a power differential at work in such a procedure and the woman is most definitely not empowered during or as a result of it. It may have an immediate effect on the perception of pain felt and so may impede the process of labour, but it may also have a longer term effect on women's libido.

When the membranes are ruptured there will be a constant flow or trickle of liquor from the woman's vagina which may be blood stained from a 'show'. Following a vaginal examination she is likely to feel damp from the lubricating jelly which has been used. This feeling may remind some women of the dampness from semen and vaginal secretions after sexual intercourse. This may be of no moment to most women they may feel merely uncomfortable with the wetness, which can be resolved by the judicious use of pads. However, others may consider it to be intolerable and a cause of great discomfort, whilst a small number may feel absolute revulsion. It certainly can be a sexual, even if not an erotic feeling, and for some may bring back unpleasant memories which can intrude on the present experience.

As the labour progresses the cervix dilates until it has been completely taken up and fully dilated. The head of the about-to-be-born baby descends and comes down through the vagina. Most women find this stage one of relief with regard to pain. The contractions have changed in character and although very strong and expulsive do not seem to be as sharply painful as before. The feeling is one of pressure into the rectum and movement of the head. This feeling, and particularly when the baby's head is coming down, into and through the vagina and pressing on the perineum is met with different reactions in women. Some welcome it almost joyfully and find a new lease of energy and push mightily. But for others the feeling of fullness and pressure feels too much to bear. As the head distends and stretches the perineum there are feelings of pain, tension, excitement, anticipation, apprehension and fear. This phase can be helped or hindered by the midwife. There are some midwives who whilst trying to be inspiring to the woman are actually being quite frightening. These are the midwives who tell the woman that she may feel as if she is about to split in two but to be reassured because she will not. These remarks are not helpful and some women report this as one of the most unpleasant memories of the second stage of labour. After all genital mutilation is a dreadful thing and one to be feared at any time by anyone. In childbirth it may be a realistic fear because many women do suffer trauma particularly to the perineum either from lacerations or from an episiotomy.

Following delivery of the baby the resemblance to the experience of orgasm is both similar and yet different. Both parents, but particularly the mother, feel relaxed (or drained) but the difference is that whilst women naturally sleep deeply after orgasm this is not the case after childbirth. The senses seem to be heightened and events are perceived more acutely, although to all outside appearance the woman looks tired out. Many women report an inability to sleep after the birth of their baby even though they may have been in labour for many hours. This is not as strange as one would think because for mammals the greatest danger to the newly-born offspring was (and is) always in the immediate period after birth so it would be perhaps more strange if women went into a deep sleep in this time.

It is hard to evaluate the effect of labour on the long-term sexuality and sexual expression of both men and women for very little definitive research has been done in this field. However there is enough in the literature to give one an idea of some of the effects of obstetric interventions. The obstetric procedures and interventions fall into two categories. There are those like vaginal examinations, artificial rupture of the membranes, and shaving and enemas (now thankfully almost obsolete practices), which in themselves are not considered by the midwives or doctors to be other than uncomfortable or embarrassing. Then there are the others such as episiotomy and perineal suturing, forceps and caesarian section which are acknowledged to be traumatic. Much of the research in this field concentrates on the long-term morbidity and physical problems such as breakdown of suturing (Ross, 1986) but there is little on the effect on libido and sexuality. However there are signs that this is changing and midwives are becoming more aware of the long term. Midwives such as Flint (1986), Sleep and Grant (1987, 1989) and Wright (1994) have drawn attention to factors which affect sexuality such as throbbing and aching of the clitoris following delivery and dyspareunia up to three months post partum which can lead to avoidance of sexual relations.

The effect of vaginal examinations has already been briefly touched upon earlier in this chapter but there are other procedures and practices in the high tech consultant units that most women deliver in which touch upon the sexuality of the women. Perhaps the first that the woman encounters is the lithotomy position. This is particularly so if the labour is to be induced. In this procedure the woman's legs are put up in stirrups and her external genitalia are completely exposed. The doctor (who in all probability is quite junior and has not met the woman before) performs a vaginal examination and using a hook of some sort ruptures the membranes. An intravenous infusion line may be set up and the woman confined to bed for the duration of the labour. If this procedure is considered at all as a negative event, then it is the dignity of the woman that is thought to be at stake. However there is much more to it than this. It touches on all sorts of cultural taboos that the person has developed during her life. The majority of women have been conditioned from early childhood to keep this part of themselves covered up. In some cultures modesty is an integral part of the shame culture and women feel shamed and degraded by the exposure of their genitals in such a manner. It says much for the resilience of women that although the experience is never forgotten, it does not traumatize or impede too much in their later lives. It could be made better though, for many doctors can perform the procedure just as easily without the use of the lithotomy poles, they just have to consider it important.

Ventouse extractions, forceps deliveries, episiotomy and suturing are other examples of procedures which can have a devastating effect on sexuality. The Ventouse apparatus is a technique whereby a vaginal examination is performed to attach a metal cup to the head of the fetus. A vacuum is built up between the cup and the fetal head and traction applied to bring the head down. It may or may not be used in conjunction with forceps. Forceps come in many different types, from the small (relatively speaking) lift out type such as Wrigley's, to the much larger and straighter Keilland's. Even the smallest look too large to be inserted into a vagina which previously has received nothing larger than a penis. Midwives and obstetricians are not unfeeling people, but they work on labour wards day in and day out and become used to these as the tools of their everyday life. The shock of seeing them for the first time has long since gone and what remains is the knowledge of how useful and lifesaving these can be. So it is not surprising that the stunning impression they have on a couple is not always appreciated by the staff. The ventouse and the forceps necessitate manipulation within the vagina which can be very uncomfortable and frightening, particularly when the life of the fetus is at stake. Episiotomy is the making of an incision to enlarge the vaginal orifice either to facilitate and protect the passage of the fetal head or to enable forceps to be inserted. It is a deep incision involving the superficial and deep layers of the muscles of the perineal body. Much of the obstetric and midwifery literature concerns itself with addressing the issues of pain and healing in the postnatal period and painful intercourse (dyspareunia) at recommencement of sexual intercourse. Very little has been published on the psychological effect on the relationship and the libido of the experience of episiotomy in its entirety.

It is hardly surprising that women have a lasting and often traumatic memory of these procedures even to feeling as if they have been raped. This is not so farfetched when one considers that the major similarity is a feeling of helplessness and loss of control, and of being done to and injured. The woman's partner can be very helpful in minimizing the effect of this situation. If he (or she) stays close to her head and 'shares her viewpoint of the birth' (Bailey, 1989) then he can be a great comfort and support, giving her an ally and a helpmeet who can help her to have some control. Staff need to be as sensitive as possible and be aware that it may not be merely a matter of expediting the procedure with as little pain as possible but that there may be more subtle and longer lasting effects at work.

Nowadays women usually do not experience labour alone, they have their partner, or a friend or relative, with them. This was met with quite a lot of opposition in the early days but has become so commonplace that not only does the midwife take the presence of the partner for granted but almost considers it essential. Kitzinger (1991) remarks that staff now consider that most of them can be 'turned into subordinate, well behaved members of the birth "team" who could be relied upon to help control the woman's behaviour, keep her calm, and make her "see reason" when staff wished to intervene or not'. Whether this point of view is valid or not is not the point, which is that men are commonplace in the modern labour ward. This being so there is another issue for the couple to consider and that is the effect of the event on the partner's future libido. It can be the most powerful and overwhelming experience ever encountered which fuses the couple together by an inseparable and life altering and enhancing bond. Or for some men it can be the greatest turn-off ever. There are many reasons for this: it may be that they feel that it was so painful for their partner that they could not subject her to it ever again, or it may be something far deeper - feelings of distress and inadequacy coupled with visions of a large and over-distended vagina can lead in a few cases to impotency in the male (Litvinoff, 1992). Midwives and obstetricians never had to consider this in the past and many would say that they do not need to now as it is out of their control and sphere of practice. This may well be true but an awareness that there is a potential problem area will lead to greater sensitivity in the treatment of men in the labour ward.

Like episiotomy, caesarian section has been the subject of much research. Also like episiotomy it has concentrated on the obviously major factors which are the indications for its performance, perinatal and maternal outcome and healing rates. Little, if anything, has ever been researched on the effect of caesarian section on a couple's sexuality and sexual function. There is evidence that it is associated with postnatal depression (Culp and Osofsky, 1989), problems of marital adjustment and difficulties with mother-infant interaction but there is nothing specific regarding its effect on sexuality. One can hazard a guess that if it has such a major effect on the dynamics of family life as a whole then there must it must be a contributory factor in their sexual relationships. Research (Kitzinger, 1991) shows that it is the loss of control over events that leaves a woman feeling disempowered, angry and depressed. Planned caesarian section is associated with less postnatal depression than is the emergency procedure. It may be that it also has a less detrimental effect on a couple's sexual function but confirmation is needed by further research.

The implications of the procedures of modern obstetrics in the aftermath of people's lives should be considered by midwives and obstetricians. Anxiety is a considerable feature of women and their partners in the surroundings of a high tech delivery suite and anxiety as Masters and Johnson (1966) pointed out as long ago as 1966 inhibits the sexual response. Strong anxiety can inhibit sexual arousal completely whilst a moderate degree of anxiety can be enough to make people feel under par and have difficulty in being aroused. If women (and men) are left with unresolved feelings of anxiety and helplessness because of the experience of childbirth, it can be transformed into problems with self-image and difficulties with their perceived sexual function. Anger, especially on the woman's part may be directed at her partner and manifest as sexual dysfunction. It behoves the professionals who work in this area to minimize the traumatic effect of such an environment as much as they can.

CHAPTER NINE

Wait Six Weeks?

No man has been a protagonist in the story,
Waiting for stitches and sleep and to be alone
And listened with tender breasts to the hesitant croak
At the bedside growing continuous as you wake,
That is the price. That is what love is worth.
                                        Lerner, A Wish

Mother or lover, can a woman be both? Or does she even want to be? These are the questions that many women after having a baby have to decide for themselves. It may have been that previously a woman was competent and in control, someone perhaps who effortlessly juggled the various demands that life made upon her. She was the efficient housewife, the expert shopper, the super organizer, the working professional and yet still found time to make her own wine, clothes, dried flower arrangements, debate the merits of post-modernism and to be a multiorgasmic lover. Well perhaps this sort of woman is very few and far between, but perhaps not so far off for many. So does something happen to a woman after having a baby which changes her in a fundamental way, and if so, is it a positive or negative change? Childbearing is a phenomenal life-changing event. One's whole life is altered and also the lives of all the family. Everyone changes roles, men and women become fathers, mothers and fathers become grandparents, kid brothers and sisters become aunts and uncles. There is a whole generation shift. It would be surprising if this proceeded uneventfully, as change is never without its ups and downs. Sexuality is a fundamental aspect of life and so must be involved in the momentous adjustments that are made by men and women on becoming parents and that change which started with the pregnancy continues in the postnatal period onwards.

The postnatal period and the puerperium are names given to the period following childbirth. The postnatal period is a legal term and very specific, i.e. it is the 28 days following the delivery during which the midwife has a legal responsibility to attend upon the mother and baby.

It used to be called the lying-in period. The puerperium on the contrary is rather less specific and is the time following childbirth during which the organs of reproduction (apart from the breasts) return to their pre-pregnant state. This is usually considered to be six weeks or 40 days. Interestingly enough this word is derived from the Latin 'puer' a boy, although after delivery of a daughter one does not have a puellaperium.

This period of time has long been associated with taboos or restrictions on sexuality. The core of the advice given to women and their partners was 'don't do it'. Much of this advice was given as if medically correct and dangers were implied if the taboo was broken. The main danger seems to be that of infection, but there has never been any evidence to substantiate this claim. Nor as far as can be determined is the infection specified. Admittedly puerperal infection was at one time not only a potential hazard but was a realistic fear and a killer. Women who were at risk of puerperal infection were at risk because of many factors not least a poor nutritional state, and delivery in a dangerous environment such as a hospital made cross-infection was a very real possibility. During the last 90 years one of the major thrusts in maternity care has been to reduce the incidence of infection, so it is not surprising that fear of introduction of organisms (e.g. E.Coli) into the vagina by the penis was considered a risk worth avoiding. However there is little data to demonstrate whether people did follow the advice given or as is usual, quietly got on with life and did their own thing.

Another reason given for abstinence in the postnatal period is the supposed danger to the reproductive organs. Again there is little or no evidence to support this in the normal course of events. However there could be danger from rough and inconsiderate sexual activity or the insertion of foreign bodies into the vagina. These actions could cause unhealed sutures to open up or the vaginal and cervical tissue to be damaged. The author did once visit a woman in her own home three days post partum to find her perineal stitches had been removed by her husband with a bread knife because they were pricking him during intercourse, but this type of behaviour is not usual.

The most probable cause of advising forbearance is a cultural inhibition. There is a deep-seated belief in many cultures that each sex is a danger to each other through contact with sexual fluids. Others believe that only one sex is in danger from the other and that is usually the man from the woman (Douglas, 1991). Sometimes the dangers are small but when associated with childbirth can be very great indeed.

Blood has always been a very potent symbol of life-threatening danger and the blood of menstruation and childbirth are greatly symbolic of danger and pollution to men. Menstrual blood because of its mystery and non-association with injury is polluting, but less dangerous than the blood of childbirth. In labour a woman went to the far boundaries of life as she and everyone around her knew full well. It is not so long ago in this country (and still remains so in many parts of the world) that a woman in labour was in very great danger of her life. In some cultures she is considered to have ventured into the spirit realm at this time. A polluting person is always a threat because they are capable, albeit unwittingly and unintentionally, of unleashing dangerous and threatening powers. To counteract these dangers various rituals are instigated, e.g. the Judaic law that forbids a man to sleep with his wife during menstruation and until she has been purified by attending the Mikvah or ritual bath. Childbirth is so polluting that in Uttar Pradesh (North India) the new mother is seen as a great danger to everyone around her and her husband in particular, so much so that she eats from separate plates which are later broken and discarded (Jeffrey, Jeffrey and Lyon, 1989). Whilst not going so far in this country there is still evidence of the danger that a woman has been in by the ceremony of Churching of women where the Priest asks the woman to give thanks:

Forasmuch as it hath pleased Almighty God of His goodness to give you safe deliverance, and hath preserved you in the great danger of childbirth. (The Book of Common Prayer, 1662)

Until relatively recently, i.e. into the 1960s, it was commonplace for women to be churched before re-entering society. In some families today elderly grandmothers will not admit a newly-delivered mother to their homes unless she has been Churched. However as a sign of the times the ceremony and its meaning have undergone a significant change. It is now a service for both parents of thanksgiving for the birth of a child and nowhere does it mention the danger of childbirth (The Alternative Service Book, 1980).

These cultural folk memories are probably more responsible for the prohibitions on sexuality in the puerperium than the advice givers are themselves aware of.

Sexuality is expressed in many ways, some of which are integral to the mother's needs at this time. It encompasses warmth and tenderness, kissing and cuddling, holding hands and being stroked. It means being loved and made to feel a sense of self-worth. It is about health and energy and vigour. A woman needs to be comforted and supported during this time and many have a very supportive partner who fulfils these needs. The most important aspect of sexual health at this time is the ability to reciprocate, and women who are able to do so are very lucky and able to pick up their lives relatively easily. The emotions that arise from being at a birth are overwhelming in their intensity and put all life's trivial worries into perspective. Men and women can feel a joy so exquisite that it is beyond words. It transforms their lives and their relationship and brings a deeper meaning and purpose. Their sex life can take on a new and altogether more fulfilling aspect as they now share an unbreakable memory bond. Couples in this situation are likely to encounter a relatively unproblematic return to harmonious sexual activity, but not always.

There are many considerations involved in the return to full sexual function after childbirth and many factors that impede progress. These fall roughly into the following categories: ritual, physical, emotional, social and contextual.

The rituals that are performed around childbirth are so central to the everyday life of a woman and so often taken for granted that they become invisible. This is particularly so in the medicalization of the postnatal period and the breeching of body boundaries that takes place. During pregnancy antenatal care is focused on the fetus to the extent that the woman's body is seen as a container for the growing fetus, to be examined and peered into all in the cause of ensuring good fetal outcome. Maternal health is monitored with the focus on factors affecting fetal health. The focus changes abruptly after birth when the mother is now examined physically with the intent of 'rubber stamping' her as fit to return to society as a mother. She is also subtly monitored for emotional and psychological fitness for motherhood. If she fails this test a case conference may be held to determine the future of her infant. This is a period of time when the power of society as employed through the 'gaze' of the institution (Foucault, 1973) is powerfully focused on the woman's body. During this time she is in a state of liminality, i.e. she is part way through a rite of passage which will return her to society as a mother for the first or second time. One of the key characteristics of a rite of passage is that the novitiate is not in control, acts in a childlike manner, is separated from her or his family and does not make decisions. This is left to the experts who organize and set the seal of approval on this process, in this case the midwives or obstetricians. Another characteristic is the refusal to see the body as having a sexual function. This can be observed in practice by the postnatal examination. The woman's genital area is exposed for inspection on a daily and sometimes twice daily basis. As Pryce (1991) observes there is an inequality in power and control between patient and carer which is seen in the symbolic and physical violation of the body in the interests of healing, and one of the inequalities is that of sexuality. In the medicalization metaphor the body is not sexual and a clinical veil is drawn, 'which screens the body from being the object of erotic desire' (*op. cit.*). It would take a brave (or deviant) woman to break away from this cultural drama and to admit openly to resuming sexual relations in the early postpartum days. In addition there would be the sheer physical impossibility of having one's partner in bed in a hospital setting even in a private room. This is despite the philosophy of care of most maternity units, which in some form or other advocates a client- centred approach with the physical, psychological and emotional needs of the woman as being the focus of the care. What couples do in the privacy of their home after a home confinement or early discharge is difficult to ascertain because the power of the institution is still manifest through the presence of the community midwife and sexuality at this time is still overtly denied.

Apart from the ritual aspects of care which mitigate against a return to sexual function there are physical factors which can cause problems to a lesser or greater degree. These include vaginal slackness, bruising and tenderness, sutures and scar tissue from caesarian section, episiotomy or laceration, haemorrhoids, lacerations of the fine mucosa around the clitoris and the labia minora, monilial infections, sore nipples and high prolactin levels. Problems with one or more of these can affect the libido.

Vaginal slackness is given little space in midwifery and obstetric textbooks and is referred to in passing as something that can be cured by pelvic floor exercises. It is true that the muscles of the pelvic floor can be returned to a good state of tone by exercise, but sometimes there is a problem which defies exercise. This is a ballooning of the vagina which occurs in some women during the missionary position and results in air being drawn into the vagina and expelled in a noisy fashion during intercourse. It is likely this is due to slight thinning of the vaginal walls and is more successfully resolved by a change in position. Another problem that seldom surfaces is that of a gaping introitus. In years past, if a woman suffered a very small tear at the mouth of the vagina it was very often left unsutured, this is not usually the case nowadays. In most women it heals satisfactorily but in some the vaginal orifice is left permanently enlarged but most importantly the muscular closure - the bulbo cavernosus muscle - is left inefficient. This results in a poor grip on the penis during sexual intercourse which leads to it being withdrawn accidently during moments of high passion - not a satisfactory situation. This could be remedied by readmission and suturing but most women prefer to leave it as it is, so alternative positions are recommended.

There is vaginal tenderness after nearly all vaginal deliveries. In some women it is manifest only as a strange awareness of the vagina and labia as being swollen and slightly uncomfortable. It is not acute enough to be considered painful but the woman is aware that there is a difference. It may also be due to the feeling of lochial discharge which is strange after months without a menstrual flow. These women are in the minority because for the majority there is some pain and tenderness. As the head descends down the vagina there is a certain amount of friction which can cause some small abrasions of the vaginal mucosa. This is more likely to occur if the membranes have been ruptured for a while. If the head descends immediately following spontaneous rupture of the membranes the gush of liquor has a lubricant effect. A forceps delivery and to a lesser extent a Ventouse delivery can lead to quite marked abrasions of the vagina and extensive bruising around the perineal area which may take quite a while to disappear. This is usually in association with the episiotomy that is part of the procedure.

Following the suturing of an episiotomy or laceration the surrounding tissue swells up and there can be pulling on the sutures. This becomes markedly worse if the suturing was performed too tightly in the first place. Not only does the swelling in itself cause discomfort but the suturing technique and the material used have a significant effect on pain and eventually dyspareunia. Findings from research into the effect of perineal trauma, its care and long term sequelae find that dyspareunia is a significant factor for many women (Sleep and Grant, 1989; Robson, 1982). This is partly due to knots of scar tissue, knots of suturing material and sometimes due to an associated vaginal dryness. reduction of the episiotomy rate and improvements in the care of perineal trauma are an ongoing feature of midwifery research.

Following a caesarean section many women are frightened to resume sexual intercourse. They fear amongst other things the weight of their partner pressing on the wound. Many imagine that they will burst open. The scar itself takes quite a while to heal, even though the uterus will be involuted back into the pelvis by the second or third week. Women complain of scar tenderness for a long time after the event and others complain of an internal pulling sensation which can be worrying, although is not usually of significance. When an emergency caesarean section has been undertaken in the second stage of labour following failed forceps, then the woman has not only an abdominal wound but a perineal wound as well, and resuming sexual relationships may just physically take longer.

Some of the problems that are considered to be minor disorders of the puerperium can hold a woman back from feeling sexually whole. Haemorrhoids is one such case. Haemorrhoids are present in nearly a third of women after delivery. They burn, they itch, they bleed and they make one's life miserable. Unfortunately, unless the woman is seen and given advice and treatment early in the postnatal period she may hang back from complaining due to embarrassment or fear. They will be spotted at the six week postnatal examination but that can be a long way off when one is in severe discomfort. Small lacerations of the friable mucosa around the clitoris and the labia minora are not usually sutured unless they are very large, and they heal up relatively quickly. However they can become bathed in urine on micturition which will sting. Kitzinger (1985) advocates the use of a witch hazel soaked pad pressed against the laceration when the woman passes urine but this is difficult to use for tears around the clitoris and urethra. Sometimes the clitoris itself may be swollen or the prepuce can be torn but this is quite rare.

A common infection after childbirth is monilia or thrush (candida albicans). It thrives when there is a change in the pH of the vagina or when antibiotics are used. So it can be quite common in postparturient women, particularly those who have had a traumatic delivery. It will cause extreme itching and discomfort to the extent that the mother's sleep is disturbed and obviously will make her feel generally under par and disinterested in sex. It can also appear on the nipples and be transmitted to or from the baby. This will make the nipples sore and perhaps crack and the woman is not likely to consider her breasts in this state as particularly wonderfully erogenous. All of these problems can be cleared up or resolved in a relatively short time but during that time they will probably reduce libido.

There are some truths and some myths surrounding breastfeeding with regard to sexuality. One of the truths is that there is a high prolactin level which has an inhibitory effect on oestrogen. It is not usually at a high enough level to dampen oestrogen sufficiently to inhibit ovulation and so theoretically should not be responsible for vaginal dryness. This is particularly so if menstruation has resumed. If a woman has dryness of the vagina she should consider using a water-based lubricating jelly as part of lovemaking, but she should also discuss it with her partner because it may be due to poor technique and lack of sensitivity during foreplay. One of the advantages of breastfeeding is that the breasts are larger and at the height of lovemaking the milk tends to flow. This can be a great turn on to both the woman and her partner during lovemaking, but for others it can have the opposite effect.

A myth, and quite a sinister one, is that women experience orgasm whilst breastfeeding. This can be frightening for people to read or hear, particularly with its connotations of incest. It is true that the effect of stimulation of the nipples causes the uterus to contract but that is all it is - a contraction. There are physiological similarities, but similarities are all that they are. The most erogenous zone in the body is the mind and women who are breastfeeding experience a very different emotion from that of sexual intercourse. This brings up a consideration of emotional factors that impede the return to a fulfilling sex life after childbirth.

The first assumption that has to be challenged is that the woman's sex life was satisfactory before pregnancy. There is a tendency to think about the childbearing woman as a stereotype, which is mid-twenties, middle-class, with a partner, and who has planned her pregnancy. Any midwife can tell you that this is not even remotely representative of the women who deliver in the average maternity unit. They range from the stereotype above through the whole range of sexually active women such as the staid married woman, the prostitute, the infertile woman pregnant after in vitro fertilization, the lesbian and the young teenager who is pregnant after her first experiments, to mention just a few. So it is easy to see how difficult it is to generalize. What is certain, however, is that many of these women will have emotional problems which either predate the pregnancy and are compounded by it or develop as a result of it. One of the shared problems for women in Western society today is a lack of confidence and self-esteem related to body image. Women are under such constant and unrelenting pressure to change and mould their bodies into an idealized shape that they become very anxious. The changes that childbirth brings can reinforce this sense of insecurity and increase the anxiety. It is a rare person that regains her figure very quickly and unchanged. A majority of women have to contend with striae gravidarum or stretch marks and these can be very upsetting. Striae are virtually ignored by the professional literature because they are of cosmetic significance only. Industry is aware of them as a potential for selling creams and lotions (which do little good). A poor perception of body image and a feeling of unattractiveness will lead to anxiety, which in itself may lead to disinterest in sex or even frigidity.

Some women (and men) suffer from emotional problems because of factors to do with the pregnancy or delivery. There may be feelings of resentment and anger because of the presence of the baby, the type of delivery, the pain suffered or the fear and helplessness engendered. One partner may view sexual intercourse as a necessary evil to be endured only as a means of getting pregnant and now it is no longer essential. If these feelings are not resolved they can lead to problems within the relationship, and particularly sexual problems. Initially it may only be sexual responsiveness that is interfered with, but if unresolved it could lead to sexual dysfunction. There are many situations that can lead to anxiety and distress, two in particular are met fairly frequently and they are the aftermath of a miscarriage or stillbirth, and the presence of a baby in the neonatal special or intensive care unit. In these cases the parents may be questioning themselves and feeling guilty and inadequate, which is not a good recipe for the resumption of the physical side of a relationship. These problems need talking out. Sometimes the father feels left out of the close relationship that develops between the new mother and her baby and he feels jealous and intrusive. This may result in him competing with the baby and being either sexually demanding or aloof and distant. Either of these two strategies will cause confusion and exhaustion in his partner.

It is vital that people in these situations are able to talk out their problems. It is a feature of marital and sexual problems that there is a lack of communication, and an open and frank discussion between couples can help resolve difficulties before they become major problems and threaten the relationship. This is not always as simple as it sounds because when there is an underlying anger or resentment it is difficult to bring out these feelings and examine them in an objective and constructive fashion. It may be that the couples are not even aware of them except on a very deep level. It is probably a good idea to discuss feelings and fears with a mature and experienced health professional or Relate counsellor who can be empathetic, non-judgemental and supportive. It may even be something that is then felt to warrant a referral to a psychosexual counsellor.

Sometimes sexual difficulties are linked to depression after childbirth. This can range from the sort of low-key depression which has been found in every longitudinal study undertaken (Najman *et al*, 1991) to a full blown psychosis. The literature on the subject of postnatal depression is extensive and it is now known that ten per cent of women referred to psychiatric clinics suffer from sexual dysfunction (Hesford and Bhanji, 1986). Another recognized feature (Chalmers, Enkin and Kierse, 1989) of postnatal depression is that it is multifactorial and is closely linked to the amount of support gained from a person's social networks.

Social and contextual factors can play a major factor in the sex life of a woman after having a baby. There are now changes in the role that each person has to assume and with it different obligations and responsibilities. There are some women who take to motherhood like a duck to water. They have a baby that feeds and sleeps well and they are surrounded by a support network of family and friends. Even so baby care is a time-consuming and demanding occupation and the tiredness that accompanies it can lead to a loss of desire. This can be made much worse if the social factors are against the woman. If she is a single parent, lonely and miles away from her family, or they are not interested, a woman can feel drained and helpless. Poor housing and struggling with poor washing and drying facilities, lack of privacy and low income can lead to suboptimal health, exhaustion and depression. It is not surprising in a case like this if the libido suffers too. These are the obvious social stresses that couples may be subject to, but here are other more everyday type situations that affect the libido. One of these is the presence of the baby itself and other children.

It is the custom in this country to have the new baby sleep in the same bedroom as its parents for a few weeks after birth. Some couples have the baby in the bed with them. While this is an excellent idea on the whole for some it may mean they cannot make love. Some couples find the presence of the baby inhibiting even if he or she is fast asleep. Others may find that their lovemaking disturbs the baby and interferes with their spontaneity. This happens to most people at some time or other and is usually met with wry resignation. It is not a problem unless it is allowed to be. There may however be simply too little time for the mother to sleep between the demands of a baby's routine wakening and her partner's lovemaking. Knowing this, she very often makes a choice and that choice is to forgo intercourse for the sake of an hour's sleep. It is not always a satisfactory solution because guilt and frustration on both sides can arise. A crying baby can lead to the man going to work worn out, so some couples end up sleeping apart at this time. It is quite common for one of them to get up in the night and go to sleep in a spare bed.

Toddlers and older children can markedly affect the sexual relationship. As every parent knows there is nothing quite so dampening to the ardour than a small voice at the bedroom door asking for a drink of water. Life can be particularly fraught if the toddler is jealous of the new baby. Many a new parent finds themselves on the edge of the bed opposite their partner with a baby, a toddler and a host of teddies between them. Older children can in their own way present another problem. It is not very easy to be spontaneous and noisily orgasmic when one's teenager is just beyond the dividing wall. Some of these problems can be rectified with a little thought before the lack of sexual intercourse becomes a habit. Parents need to make their bedroom a haven for themselves and try to make the children understand that it is a private area, and beds can be moved away from adjoining walls. However there may still be a problem of role conflict. Some people, women in particular, have the idea that a mother must be a madonna figure rather than a lover and so must lose all interest in sex. Obviously this is not and should not be the case, but people have to work at their relationship at this time. It is a good idea if they can get a babysitter and get dressed up and go out for an evening. If this is not possible due to lack of babysitters or finances they could make a night in for themselves and make it a special event. The woman can get made up and perhaps they could have a bottle of wine and a meal by candlelight with soft music playing in the background, or whatever it is that will make it special for them.

The final ingredient in this brew of anxiety and sexual turn offs is contraception. Anxiety, as has been noted is a major cause of poor sexual responsiveness and even sexual dysfunction, and a major anxiety for healthy fertile couples is the threat of an unwanted pregnancy. It is imperative that they use not only an effective method of contraception but one that is acceptable and user friendly. The midwife and the general practitioner will both be happy to give advice in the early postnatal period and the woman can be referred or refer herself to a family planning advisory centre. The address of the nearest clinic can be found in the Yellow Pages under 'Clinics'.

CHAPTER TEN

The Midwife as Self

Self reverence, self knowledge, self control,
These three alone lead life to sovereign power.
Tennyson, Oenone.

Midwives are human! Sometimes this is forgotten by the public, sometimes by midwifery managers and sometimes by midwives themselves. Midwives as a breed are a very professional group of people and pride themselves on leaving their own problems 'at the door'. They change into acting role as they change into uniform, but most have already internalized the concept and feel themselves to be midwives through and through. This is so intrinsic that it is very rarely examined or questioned. It is as natural as any other role in life. Midwives are mothers, fathers, wives, husbands, lovers, aunts, uncles, students, teachers, staff midwives, E grades, and sisters, to name but a few titles or positions. These are labels and a label only becomes a role when 'rights, norms, duties and responsibilities (are) attached to it' (Cowling *et al*, 1988). The role holder does not create the role unaided, it is a team effort with others, the members of the 'role set' (Merton, 1970). Members of a role set have specific expectations of how role holders within that set should behave and for the most part role holders conform to the expectations. This is due to two factors: first the role holder has taken on the beliefs, values and assumptions of the role over a considerable time and has internalized them. Secondly, failure to conform to the role set's expectations will lead to conflict and probable expulsion of the role holder from the group. This is a perfectly natural feature of group behaviour. All groups have norms to which their members conform. If an individual has a problem adapting he or she will be isolated and frozen out, expelled from the group or leave voluntarily and the group's internal equilibrium will be reinstated (Sherif, 1936). Sometimes a phenomenon termed role-conflict occurs, which is when the individual either finds that members of the role set has differing expectations in relation to the person's role or that she has two or more roles which are in conflict. This leads to role stress, a psychological reaction to role conflict which impairs the mental and physical well-being of the person (Cooper and Davidson, 1992).

There are two key responsibilities to the role of a midwife. The first is implicit in the meaning of the word midwife, 'with woman'. This holds that the woman and her needs are the central focus of the care given. The second is a responsibility to give non-judgmental care, regardless of the midwives own personal values and beliefs. In the main, this is not too heavy a load for midwives and most successfully achieve a balance between their inner and outer persona. The major issues of conflict, such as abortion, are usually satisfactorily resolved by the midwife in question referring the woman to another midwife for any particular advice whilst still retaining the duty to care.

There are, however, parts of a midwife's life experience which may well impinge on her role, sometimes even without her conscious awareness. One of these is her sexuality. Childbirth in itself is a sexual event as has already been discussed in Chapter 8 and is the result of a sexual act. This makes it a different and unique work experience from most people's - even nurse's. How the midwife handles herself in the face of this depends on three factors, her training, her role models and her own attitudes to sexuality.

Despite its importance, the issues surrounding sexuality have not been addressed until relatively recently in the training and education of midwives. In fact there have been midwifery tutors in this author's experience who were so inhibited in the discussion of sexual matters that they, for instance, could teach the male reproductive system without mentioning the word penis, would ensure that the models of the breasts were turned inwards in glass cupboards so as not to offend, and would not teach family planning at all. However such teachers were in the minority , but nevertheless the subject itself was scantily dealt with even in textbooks for midwives.

Midwives had to fall back on role models for their style and so professional attitudes were perpetuated. This was usually to the benefit of the women and their families. Most midwives have fond memories of particular midwives who were role models for them, midwives who cared for the woman and her partner in a calm, comforting, non-intrusive way. They can also recall the midwives who were a role model in a different way. These were the midwives that one hoped one would never be like. Apart from their personal influence on a one-to-one basis they could have quite wide reaching effects. Sometimes a negative attitude, particularly from a senior midwife with power and authority, could endow the culture of the particular maternity unit with an atmosphere that was not conducive to the best possible experience for women. Take, for example, the case of a unit where some of the senior midwives had an apparent distaste for the presence of men in the labour wards, and ascribed to them prurient motives for being with their partners. This engendered a sense of anger, powerlessness and role-conflict in the less senior midwives and a furtiveness to their efforts to accommodate the families wishes. It also went into the folklore of the surrounding community that the experience of childbirth in that unit was not pleasant for men. Luckily this type of attitude to care is in the past and would not be tolerated by the Trust management of today.

However, if one defines sexuality as encompassing one's deepest longings, as Hogan (1980) does and as Watson (1991) says, is 'all that being a female or a male is to a person and that the expression of sexuality is a continuous need to convey that meaning to others' then it becomes clear that being a midwife cannot be a sexually neutral role. This is not to say the midwife's sexuality is actively expressed as a part of the care but rather that her values, beliefs and attitudes to sexuality will have an effect on the care she gives and the way she relates to women and their partners. Very little work has been done in this area and so rather than make sweeping generalizations it is perhaps preferable to bring some of the differences in midwives' sexual attributes to the reader's attention as a starting point for reflection.

Midwives are as different in sexual attributes as they are in shape, size, height and colouring. For a start there are now gender differences, because there has been a steady trickle of men into the profession since the early 1980s, although the majority of midwives are still women. Each person has their own gender ascription and methods of sexual expression and whether they are satisfied with it or not is a personal matter for them alone, except that is if it impinges on the care they give. Midwives can be found as virgins or experienced lovers. They can be heterosexual or homosexual. The women can be, and often are mothers themselves, or they may be childless and yet fertile, childless and hoping to conceive, childless and infertile, or they may be menopausal or post-menopausal. The men also may be parents, and indeed fatherhood may be the triggering factor for their initial interest in midwifery.

It is quite wrong and foolish to ascribe behaviour patterns and motivation on people merely on their attributes, but it is worth considering the problems that individuals may have to deal with, such as the virgin midwife. It is rare nowadays for young people in their 20s to be virgins and so this in itself sets the midwife apart experientially from the mothers she is dealing with. It may be that she is a virgin for any number of reasons. It could be that it is part of her cultural upbringing and/or religious beliefs that she does not have sex outside marriage and she is not married yet. She may be a nun. She may have not met a man that she wants to go to bed with or wants to go to bed with her. Or she may be disinterested in or actively dislike men or the idea of sexual intercourse. Each of these may make her view the mother and her partner differently. The last reason apart, the effect on her caregiving will probably be just a lack of depth to the insight she has on the process. Except perhaps if religious and moral attitudes cause her to be judgemental about single mothers. One major area of disadvantage to the midwife of being a virgin or a non-mother for that matter, is in the delivery of a parentcraft sessions. The planned aspect is easy enough, but when it comes to the spontaneous question and answer sessions, particularly on contraception methods and tips about babycare the midwife can feel disadvantaged. However, this is not the case if the midwife has good group facilitation skills and can enable the parents to learn from each other's experiences. If she has a problem with men it may spill over into the care. Communication is not merely about information. It takes place through the subtleties of body language which can communicate an attitude as much or more that any words can. This will prove to be a block and a barrier in all the care she gives to childbearing women and their partners. Midwives are in a powerful position over the women and this is particularly the case in the labour ward, and some of this power can be directed towards the partner in very subtle ways such as withholding of information. Also, as was pointed out earlier, it can have very serious effects on the service as a whole if such a person has a measure of institutional power.

For a midwife, being an experienced heterosexual lover is probably the least problematic state to be in, except that it may make the person see herself as 'normal' and anybody who differs from this as abnormal. If this is so there is a danger that she may not recognize that people have a right to different ways of sexual expression. This may lead to difficulties in recognizing women with different needs. Or it may give rise to judgemental attitudes to people, such as lesbian couples who fall outside her definition of normality. Again this would not be too significant in practice except for the power that midwives do hold. For example, lesbian couples may be under greater scrutiny as parents by carers who will undoubtedly have the welfare of the baby at heart but may not always be able to recognize their own prejudice.

Many midwives are homosexual and whilst some have 'come out', many still have not, which is a great pity for it must be very difficult and feel very unsupported to deny one's sexuality. Lesbians have a great deal to offer as midwives, for after all it is a female dominated profession caring for other females. There can be a great feeling of solidarity and sisterhood with a strong pro-woman element to delivery of care. The feminist view can mitigate against the patriarchal power of medical domination and act as a watchdog on behalf of a woman-centred approach. Just as a female nurse working with male patients is a professional person who is not going to make overtures to the men, so the lesbian midwife is not going to behave other than impeccably with the women. However they must suffer, or feel that they will suffer from prejudice or marginalization, otherwise more would feel comfortable about being frank about their sexuality. In many ways their fears are not unfounded, because the difficulty that the midwifery profession has to face as a whole is that of being a majority of women, and as such disempowered in the hierarchy. Any midwife who is very assertive and outspoken is at risk of having her femininity questioned, which is a very culturally stereotypical response indeed! The only problem that a lesbian midwife might have that interferes with care is if she, like the examples cited above, does not like men. This is not a common feature of lesbianism and must not be thought to be.

Being a mother oneself was at one time, and still is, in some cultures, one of the necessary qualifications to being a midwife. There is no doubt that there are many positive advantages to being a mother as a midwife. Having personally undergone the experience can lead to greater awareness and understanding of the process and the woman's needs. It gives another dimension to the nature of the work and an insight that can never be gained from observation or books. Many a midwife has commented to this author how much their practice has changed since they have had their own children. Pain seems to be the topic which provides the most insight. As one midwife commented, 'I always knew that labour was painful but I never imagined it could be that bad until I had my own baby. Now I know what pain is really like'. They also know what it feels like to become rather vulnerable and scared of not being able to cope with a baby or to panic at the slightest hint of danger to the baby. Motherhood gives the midwife a point of reference that is particularly unique to women just as is menstruation. It makes her an equal and a member of `the club' which can be very useful to women particularly in labour. It seems to be particularly comforting for women in labour to talk to their midwife about her experience of giving birth. It seems to be reassuring on two counts, first, that the midwife can understand what she is going through, and secondly, that it is a normal process with a good outcome at the end of it.

Midwives who do not have children would say that it does not affect the way they give care because just like a nurse one does not need to have had a major operation to care for a surgical patient, and this is undoubtedly true. However it does seem to be that women on the whole seem to prefer the midwife to be a mother. There can be a negative aspect to the midwife's own experience of motherhood for a number of reasons. A midwife who has had a very difficult delivery, perhaps after a prolonged and painful labour, may not be as sympathetic to women who she perceives are not suffering as much as she did. Or the opposite may have happened, she may have had a very easy experience of childbirth and secretly feels that women who complain are rather 'soft'. This type of feeling may lead to brusqueness in dealing with the women or at best a lack of tenderness and compassion.

In the postnatal period midwives own experiences of feeding may colour the advice they give to new mothers. This is particularly true of breastfeeding. If a midwife finds it inherently distasteful, or she has difficulty in touching another woman's breasts, then her advice and care may be less than ideal. If she passionately wanted to breastfeed herself but could not for some reason or another then old unresolved feelings may surface and be a hindrance to good communication at this time. It may be that she breastfed very successfully and has the zeal of a missionary in its promotion, to the extent that she even unwittingly pressurizes the woman rather than advising her. (This obsession with breastfeeding can also be found in some nulliparous midwives.) Breastfeeding and its promotion does not seem to be a neutral topic which is concerned merely with the best way of feeding a baby. It is value laden and highly emotive and is bound up with the sexuality of women.

It is highly likely that all childless midwives will, at some time or another, feel a pang of longing at the sight of a new baby. Their brand new, helpless, vulnerable, beauty has an appeal that touches most human hearts. For midwives who are childless by choice this may well be just a passing desire or one that they defer until later in their lives and it does not impinge on their care in an obvious way. For midwives who are infertile, or for perimenopausal or post-menopausal midwives it may bring more lasting problems. To be trying, unsuccessfully, to have a baby can be very emotionally upsetting, but to work with babies day in and day out can almost be like rubbing salt in the wounds. This is particularly so if the mothers of the babies are both apparently super fertile and disinterested in motherhood. There are such mothers in every maternity unit, people who have several children one after another with an apparent disregard for their welfare. Most midwives, and this includes infertile midwives, are able to conform to the group norm of professional and non-judgemental care, but occasionally bitterness spills over into the professional life and can be manifest as super politeness and a cold efficiency. Perimenopausal midwives come face to face with their ticking biological clock everyday when they see new mothers and babies. Most of them are very motherly to the women and bring their mothering skills into play as part of the care they give. However for some it makes them slightly reckless and the author knows of several midwives of this age who have played 'Russian roulette' with their method of contraception. This feeling usually passes and the midwife comes to terms with these feelings until she either becomes pregnant with all the sequelae that accompanies motherhood in later life, or she gains the safe haven of post-menopause.

The important point to all these issues surrounding the sexual status of midwives is that they become aware of their feelings. Not only should they be aware, they should examine them in depth and gain insight and development from the examination. The important thing is to bring the strengths of their situation to the care they give and most importantly not to become embittered in any way. Some enlightened senior midwifery managers are aware of the stressful nature of the work that midwives do, particularly where a stillbirth has occurred and so are introducing counselling services as part of the staff support system. These are usually run by professional and confidential counsellors and could provide a midwife who has a problem relating to the women in her care, due to her own sexual circumstances, the ideal opportunity to offload and grow.

Male attendants have gradually and consistently made their presence felt in midwifery from the 1700s and the fact has been well-researched (McKenna, 1991). Men had been admitted to the profession as a result of Barbara Castle's (the then British Secretary of State) Sex Discrimination Act of 1975. The profession had found it hard to accept on the grounds as put forward by the Royal College of Midwives that:

1. Midwives gave intimate care to women and the majority of the public would not accept this care from a man.

2.   The desired psychological support required during pregnancy is best given by a female.

3.   The fact that the midwife is a woman is an important part of her function.

During the 1980s there was a great interest in the presence of males in midwifery (McKenna, 1991). There was much debate in the nursing and midwifery press with supporters putting forward the case that mothers do not object because they do not see the difference between male general practitioners, male obstetricians and male midwives (Speak and Aitken-Swan, 1982). Their opponents did not accept this position and some quoted husbands as being against male midwives being with their wives (Moore, 1982). There is an immediate, and not always obvious, difficulty with the studies into the acceptability of men in the profession and they are: first, that a male bias may be present, and secondly, the problem of the subordinate status of women in Western society (Walton, 1993). According to Moore (1988) this is manifest not at the level of empirical research but at the theoretical and analytical level which means that analytically women are invisible. This is a problem of muting and is at the level of frustrated communication. Men and women have different world views and models of society. Muting is:

> refracted through and embedded in many different
> social spaces: in seating arrangements, economic
> patterns, status, value and symbolic systems, and
> so forth (Dube, Leacock and Ardener, 1986).

The phenomenon of men speaking for or representing women causes no comment because of the patriarchal social context within which women live and work.

As a result of the dearth of good solid research into the matter and the very small numbers of males in midwifery it is difficult to discuss the effect of their sexuality on care without seeming prejudiced either in favour or against. It is interesting, however, that a representatively large number of males in midwifery at the present time have self-selected themselves away from the giving of direct intimate to women. They have management positions or are in 'safe' areas like the neonatal unit. There may be various reasons for this, ambition, for instance, but it may point to an underlying feeling of vulnerability. If this is the case (and it may well not be) then it may have sad repercussions for the type of care women receive. It has already been pointed out that some female midwives have difficulty in handling women's breasts. If this is the case with male midwives then it may detract from their ability to give 'hands on' care to women. They may also be vulnerable when practising as a community midwife. (They would not be unique in this as other health professional groups such as health visitors or community psychiatric nurses face similar potential problems without apparent difficulty.) It seems to be that the three points put forward by the Royal College of Midwives (see previous pages) have still not been researched properly. Until now the research, such as it is, has concentrated on point 1, i.e. that the public would not accept care from a man. The other two, regarding the gender of the midwife as being a positive factor in the care, have been virtually ignored.

Perhaps gender is not too important a factor in the giving of midwifery care because it is the membership of the group and conformity to group norms that acts as a standard setting device and a means of channelling the power of the institution, and this power is always patriarchal and male dominated. Midwives do not possess power within their own right and this is obvious in many ways. One of the significant characteristics of a profession is that it defines its own parameters of practice. For instance, the medical profession takes cogniscance of modern developments such as the growing interest in alternative therapies and takes them on board or not as the case may be, but the important feature is that it is answerable in this matter only to its own regulating body. This is not so for midwifery. Other professions are instrumental in the definition of the midwife's role, e.g. the prescription that midwives can only deal with the 'normal' and the definition of what that normal is. Midwives at whatever level they practice work with delegated power.

This can be seen quite clearly in the labour ward (Walton, 1993) where the midwife gives the bulk of the day-to-day care and is responsible for a vast amount of decision-making. She also has authority over the house officers who she directs towards the women needing attention, gently guides them in many procedures, and even gives them permission to leave the ward. When a registrar is about to leave the labour ward he may ask the permission of the senior sister but it is done in a very different way, often jokingly, as if to reinforce the role differential, and consultants do not ask to leave at all, they will make a remark such as, 'is there anyone else you would like me to see before I go'. This setup is very similar to a traditional household in male dominated societies where women rule the roost and have authority over all the household including the teenage boys until the men arrive home. Then the boys join the men and the women have no power over them. This is the case with the house officers. However junior and inexperienced they are, they will join the ranks of the doctors when the registrar or consultant is on the scene.

The lack of empowerment of midwives is seen in the use of space in the labour ward. The bulk of the space is normally used by the midwife. She is free to move around in it and organize its usage, whereas the woman and her partner are not. However when the doctor is called in the space becomes his or hers and the midwife acts as an assistant. It is also seen in the control of methods of pain relief. The midwifery profession is not able to take the initiative in the use of pain relief. Midwives are hedged in by cautions and restrictions from other professions. This is particularly evident in the administration of pain relief and has been so from the days of the witch hunts when midwives were prohibited from using herbs and potions. Even something as simple as TENS, which is so safe that the mothers can buy or hire and use it themselves, is sanctioned for administration by midwives. Although they can use pethidine in certain circumstances on their own responsibility this is limited and circumscribed in such a way as to leave very little room for flexibility in decision-making. This, along with other drug administration, is controlled by the medical profession who fiercely guard their authority to prescribe. Ann Oakley (1990) considers this power to be not only patriarchal but misogynous and she (p.255) quotes Margaret Mead's observation that,

Men began taking over obstetrics and they invented a tool (the vaginal speculum) that allowed them to look inside women. You could call this progress, except that when women tried to look inside themselves it was called practising medicine without a license (Mead, 1974) .

Even though male midwives may be included by doctors in more of the decision-making (even when very inexperienced) (Walton, 1993), it is highly unlikely that the balance of professional power will change in the near future, and even male midwives will still be working, as are the female midwives, with delegated authority. Even if their numbers increase dramatically it is still the group that sets the norms. The gender and sexuality of its members whilst still relevant is not as potent an ingredient as the external forces on influencing the provision of care.

PART FOUR

Sexuality, Problem or Passion?

CHAPTER ELEVEN

The Survivor

Men fashioned the image of chance as an excuse for their own
thoughtlessness; for chance rarely fights with wisdom, and a man of
intelligence will by foresight, set straight most things in his life.
Democritus (Barnes, 1987)

Being pregnant and having a baby is always a stressful event, even when everything is socially well, the mother's and the fetus's health are good and the baby is wanted. These are the criteria that occupy most people's minds and if they are fulfilled the pregnancy and labour is considered to be 'low risk'. Stress, if considered at all, will also be thought of as minimal. However there is a group of women who may fulfil all the criteria but for whom childbirth will not only be stressful but potentially abusive, frightening and painful. These are women who are abuse survivors. Abuse can be physical or sexual or both and in America it is estimated that one in every 50 pregnant women may be the subject of domestic violence (Bohn, 1990). Obviously this is not a socially healthy situation and whilst representing an overwhelming problem that must be tackled in order to help women and their children and to prevent the cycle recurring, it is not one that will be considered here, except to say that it is, like sexual abuse, one of many strategies that an abuser uses to exert power over his (or her) victim. What is of concern when focusing on sexuality is sexual abuse, its survivors and the professional care givers in the maternity services.

There are many people working as midwives or doctors who on an intellectual level know that, statistically, the women that they care for must contain a significant number of people who have been sexually abused as children. Some estimates put the figure at one in ten of the population (Draucker, 1992) but it may be much higher, for how can it be truly quantified? Some of the survivors are themselves unaware of what has happened until they recall or flashback and perhaps some never will. The abuse may be locked into their subconscious and even into their muscles so firmly that it is hidden in a place that the mind will not venture until another abusive situation causes it to be unlocked, sometimes with devastating consequences. Why it is that midwives and doctors can know on a cognitive level that these women exist, but fail to recognize them or their existence in practice is something that has not been fully explored as yet but may have something to do with the type of care practices that exist in obstetrics and midwifery. Not only are they intimate procedures but in some cases may mimic abuse in itself and so it may be that for care givers who have a positive self-image and concept of the care that they provide, the thought that they may be identified as perpetrators of abuse is too farfetched to even contemplate. Nevertheless this is not the case for everyone, for there are professionals such as midwife Lynn Baptisti Richards (1992) who maintains that,

We continue to accept sexual and mental abuse of birthing women as 'just the way birth is'. Abuse at birth is the norm. Whilst this may be too strong for many to stomach it is nonetheless a viewpoint that must be considered for the women's sake. They have suffered enough already.

The woman's first meeting with the midwife and the obstetrician is usually in early pregnancy. She either goes to the maternity unit or is visited in her home by the midwife and a detailed history taken. This usually includes questions about her physical and mental health, past and present medical and surgical history, family history, social history and most importantly her past and present obstetric history. In this way her problems both present and potential may be identified and her care planned accordingly. Although it has been recommended (Courtois, 1988; Bohn, 1990) that women should be assessed for abuse in their relationships past or present, it is not part of the routine of British antenatal history taking. Without a sensitive and aware approach it is unlikely that a woman will volunteer the information unaided, although she may give hints. There are many clues that the woman may be giving out and one such is the expression of fear about the forthcoming delivery. Most women have some feelings of apprehension about giving birth but sexual abuse survivors may be more apprehensive than most. They may also report difficulty in sleeping, or report having unusual dreams or nightmares. A sensitive and skilful midwife can use the antenatal history session as a stepping stone to forming a personal relationship that enables the woman to explore her fears in a safe environment and empowers her to speak. Empowerment is a quality of life that sadly is very often lacking for these women for they have been victimized, laden with guilt and been deprived of the emotional nurturing which is essential for sexual well-being and self-esteem.

During pregnancy the woman is the recipient of antenatal care. Many writers, Oakley (1990) in particular, have drawn attention to the paternalism of the medical profession and to the infantilization of women (Kirkham, 1989). Women are treated like children and spoken to as such. They are told to 'pop off' their knickers and to 'hop' on to couches and are called sweetie, lovey, petal, queen and princess. When they comply with the instructions they are told they are 'a good girl'. For most women these attempts to reduce them in status are highly irritating but nothing more. For women who have been abused it can feel more sinister. One of the many unpleasant aspects of abuse is the helplessness and vulnerability of the victim. This leads many of the women to be very anxious about being in control and being treated as an adult. This is extremely important to them and to be talked down to, in however a well-meaning way, is damaging. As one woman said,

All through my care I have been treated as a child......What he [the doctor] was trying to do was take my choice from me and I think that's where I felt it is abusive, about taking control, trying to inflict your views and wants on another person. (Walton, 1993)

The procedures that are part of antenatal care can be very threatening and feel like an abusive situation. Women are still in some units routinely made to remove their underwear before seeing the doctor. This makes one feel very vulnerable (and is quite unnecessary). They are then abdominally and vaginally examined whilst lying on a couch staring at a ceiling. Fingers are inserted into their vaginas. Cold hard speculum are used (think what this is like for someone who has been abused with a bottle or some such implement). Doctors look into vaginas but not always at faces. As one woman said, it was as if the doctor was looking at a body and performing a procedure but not thinking of her as a person going through the process. As Jenny Kitzinger (1992) points out, it replicates abuse where children have endured physical intrusion, lost control over their bodies, suffered voyeurism and have been totally powerless and vulnerable.

On consideration it is easy to highlight the obvious procedures that may be distressing for abuse survivors but it is not so easy to pinpoint the more subtle ways in which the feelings can flood back. This is because sexual abuse survivors are a minority within a minority. Women are, as Beauvoir (1975) points out, the second sex. They are muted in society and do not have the language of the dominant sex, their free expression is blocked at the level of ordinary, direct language (Ardener, 1975). So situations which are part of the everyday experience of women are not featured as particularly damaging or hurtful. This includes depersonalized antenatal care where women sit and wait to be seen by a midwife whom they have never met before and are not likely to meet again. It includes not having real choices and no say in the process at all. This silence from women is all the more sad because in abusive situations the abuser has always managed to keep the child silent. Midwifery care is in the process of being changed, and authentic, individualized care will hopefully become a reality for more and more women. It has come about as a result of pressures from within and without the midwifery profession and will perhaps enable women's voices, including those of the survivors, to be heard.

Despite the changes that are being made in the care of pregnant women there are still situations that are stressful to women and sexual abuse survivors in particular. One of these is the determination of the medical profession to 'see' the fetus. A huge industry underpins the obsession with making the uterus more transparent and the fetus more visible. It is a rare woman who goes through her pregnancy without at least one obstetric ultrasound surveillance. This procedure is hurtful to the survivor on two counts. One is that it is physically uncomfortable and restraining, which is not usually considered to be significant, but to be lying down, with a full bladder and to have one's abdomen pressed is not a good feeling. It is also not a physiologically advantageous position for either the mother or the fetus, causing, as it does, the gravid uterus to press against the inferior vena cava and a resulting reduction in the oxygen supply to both the maternal and the fetal brain. The second is that one is not in control of the event and, in fact, is of secondary importance being reduced to a uterus on view. As Ian Donald (1969), the obstetrician responsible for the introduction of ultrasound into obstetrics, so tellingly reveals, the mother has been considered an iron curtain which has now been swept away. She is now truly invisible as a person and this does not go unnoticed by the women themselves. It depersonalizes and disempowers them. It also controls them. As Anne Oakley (1990) (p. 185) points out, by enabling mothers to see their fetuses doctors can now encourage early bonding and in fact 'antenatal care has finally discovered mother love' which can now be 'added to the repertoire of reproductive activities named and controlled by obstetricians'.

The process of pregnancy and childbirth can be considered as a rite of passage where the woman is the initiate. One of the features of a rite of passage (Van Gennep, 1960) is that there is a social drama taking place which is characterized by a sense of mounting crisis with the initiate being more and more liminoid. (Liminality (Turner, 1974) is a state during which a person's social relationships are different from those that are part of their everyday world. In this situation people who would not normally associate with each other are thrown together because of circumstances.) That this mounting crisis is a reality for sexually abused women is confirmed by Rose (1992), who relates that she was totally unaware of being sexually abused until she was six months pregnant with her first child and had subsequent flashbacks in labour. Another significant aspect of a rite of passage is that the initiate is expected to assume the behaviour and status of a small child prior to redressive action and reintegration into society. This is very difficult for sexual abuse survivors for as one woman said having an element of control was very important to her. For her the making of a birth plan which stated categorically that no intervention would take place without her having been consulted was all part of this.

Labour is a particular time of fear for the sexual abuse survivor. There are all sorts of fears starting with the fear of being found out. Many women have spent all their lives living with their 'secret' and their guilt and shame because the perpetrators are very good at putting the onus on the children to make them feel that they are to blame, that they are dirty and bad. The survivor is often left with a feeling of not being 'normal' because they were abused and because of how they reacted or did not react to the abuse (Gillespie, 1993). This fear of being found out can have led to their inability to be open and bring the matter to the attention of anyone, even their partners, although as has been said they may be giving out clues that indicate distress and a need to talk. The threat of exposure and the need to be in control may affect the attitude of such a woman to pain relief. It may be that she is adamant that she will not have anything under any circumstances and sticks to this decision in the face of all odds. Or it may be that she will choose something like an epidural that leaves her mentally clear. Or she may go to the opposite extreme and ask for a general anaesthetic that puts her out of the situation completely.

There are all sorts of aspects of labour that may be a strain for the woman. Enemas on admission are not part of modern care in labour but may be offered in certain circumstances, for instance if the rectum is loaded and impacted. This may constitute quite a trial for the woman but she should be able to refuse it. The trouble is that often she may not feel she has the power to refuse, or that a refusal will bring more attention to herself when she just wants to be inconspicuous. There is another side to this as well. There are women who would like an enema, not for itself, but because they are so afraid of being 'dirty' that they cannot bear the thought of soiling the bed at delivery. They have a dilemma, because asking for one may make them noticed and perhaps thought of as odd, but not having one may make them extremely anxious and hold back in labour.

There can be a problem regarding wetness in labour. This can be caused by seepage of amniotic fluid when the membranes are ruptured or from the lubricating gel used as part of the vaginal examination. For some women the wet or slimy feeling is an extremely unpleasant sensation which stirs up old memories of abuse. Some men have taken delight in humiliating their victims by soiling them with body fluids and this feeling of revulsion may be overwhelming to the woman. She may be absolutely adamant that she has a dry pad to the extent that the midwife may consider that she is being obsessive.

Induction of labour, Ventouse extraction or forceps procedures can be a nightmare for the woman. Her legs are up in stirrups and there are strangers in the room. She may feel that once again she is being objectified and depersonalized. Old feelings of being the subject of voyeurism may well surface. This is not helped by the set up of many obstetric units where the procedures are performed by staff that the woman may have never met before and who in their own way are distancing themselves by the assumption of a professional persona.

Then there are the tools, the equipment, those huge, cold, hard forceps being thrust so inexorably into the vagina, the round hard cup of the Ventouse, and the hand which remorselessly wrestles inside her. Couple these with the pain of labour, focused on the genitals and it is little wonder that women who have been abused flash back to the situation of their childhood and for some of them the reaction is the same. They may become timid, quiet, compliant and dissociate. Dissociation is common for abuse survivors, they disappear from the situation. As Anna Rose (1992) describes it, it is a means of escaping, of being somewhere else and of viewing the scene as if from the ceiling. This is not a good way of coping because it puts the woman back into the past and into the vulnerable situation. She needs to be helped to remain focused, to be in the present, to be empowered to act as an adult, and to make her own decisions. Midwives who speak baby talk take heed!

The opposite may be true - the woman may not be quiet and compliant. She may have successfully dissociated herself from the traumas of her childhood to the extent of burying it deeply in some far corner of her mind. As one survivor said (McNamara, 1989) she had decided long ago 'to forget it, never speak of it, never even think of it'. Unfortunately the woman may return to the abuse with a vengeance in labour particularly if the pain becomes too bad to bear or when the head is distending the vagina and the perineum. It may feel just like the original violation and it may cause her to panic, to lose control and to be hysterical. She particularly needs a caring sensitive midwife at this time.

After the baby is born the woman may need perineal suturing, and this should be done by someone who has looked after her in her labour and ideally not with her legs supported by lithotomy poles. Apart from the problems of voyeurism that have already been mentioned, it is worth the professional being aware that some children have been tied to bed posts as part of the abuse and so having one's legs in stirrups is yet another reminder of the helplessness that was once felt.

Breastfeeding may not be an issue for some women because the breasts not having been developed as a child were not an issue in the abusive situation. For other women they may have fears about their adequacy as a mother and their ability to protect their child and difficulties with breastfeeding may arise because of it. These feelings will not be helped by some writers' views that breastfeeding is an erotic experience. This may be particularly the case with the mothers of boy babies. They may also fear changing or bathing their babies or letting anyone else do so. Another issue for the survivor is the feeling of inadequacy and low self-esteem that has been part and parcel of her life to date. It may lead her to feel that she is both unworthy and incapable of being a good mother. This feeling may, in fact, be reinforced by her partner, for she may have not had enough self-esteem to have chosen a supportive partner.

Postnatal depression may be linked to these feelings of inadequacy, poor self-image and esteem which may be compounded by health professionals who miss the clues and in their concern for the baby reinforce these feelings of unworthiness. Along with these worries may be fear of having the baby taken away from her if she 'tells', so the feelings of depression, shame and guilt continue and so does the secrecy, until perhaps a crisis occurs or a perceptive health professional enables, facilitates and gives the woman permission to speak of her experiences.

Midwives are not in the main trained counsellors, nor should they be, for counselling, particularly with the survivor of abuse, is a specialized field requiring an individual and probably lengthy therapeutic relationship. What midwives must be is aware, sensitive, accepting and non-judgemental. They need awareness combined with knowledge.

It is important that they have some information either before or after registration regarding child sexual abuse and most importantly its effects on adult survivors. They need to know that child sexual abuse is a fact and that it is not confined to one social class or grouping. It occurs in every stratum of society and it is characterized by secrecy. Breaking the taboo and bringing its existence into the open can help many women to accept that the past was not their fault. (Incidentally it may be useful for organizations dedicated to helping children to realize this, and slogans which imply that a child has the power to say no, are not always helpful either to the child at risk or to the general population's understanding of the power dynamics at work.)

Midwives should be aware that many of the women they care for will be sexual abuse survivors and they should be alert for the clues that such women are giving out (or demonstrate, such as old genital or rectal scars). Midwives should try to make the history taking and antenatal examination sessions times of low stress, openness and empathy. This can be achieved by ensuring that there is privacy and sound proofing and enough time to enable the formation of a safe and trusting relationship which will help the woman to disclose her fears and perhaps the reasons behind them. This will not happen until midwives truly understand the nature and importance of these sessions and are strong enough to challenge managerial assumptions of work throughput. If women do disclose their experiences and require further help midwives should be knowledgeable about the resources available in the community to help and support them. If these are limited they should, as a profession, lobby for more.

Midwives who give antenatal education are in a position to do two things that may help. The first is to bring the subject up in the first place, perhaps as part of a discussion group with questions and answers. This will be particularly useful if the participants know that they can contact the midwife privately for further exploration or help. The second is that she can be aware, as Simkin (1992) points out, that survivors may be resistant to lying down and relaxing among strangers. In fact she may be too tense to lie down. Watching films of birth or listening to phrases which echo dominance by a male, e.g. teaching the partner to 'coach' or control her may evoke panic type reactions. If the midwife notices anything like this she may try to follow it up in a sensitive manner rather than dismissing the woman in some way.

It is important that midwives are not judgemental and do not put women into mental categories of being over anxious and fuss pots, nuisances or demanding. As has been mentioned, probably the most important aspect of their care for such women is the necessity to remain in control. This may lead to the formulation of care plans that must be adhered to, or the necessity to have long and detailed explanations about their care or the condition of their fetus. As one woman said (Walton, 1993) when describing the way she had had to make a fuss to get professional information that would enable her to make a decision about the pregnancy, 'he didn't treat me as an adult who was making a very difficult decision'.

Being in control and being empowered to make decisions is very important and so is trust. To many of the women trust is very important and so midwives should ensure that if something has been agreed, for example as part of a birth plan, it should never be altered or deviated from without discussion with the woman. They should also make a great effort not to speak down to women or their partners in any way. Often it is done with the best intentions, probably because midwives muddle up caring for women with caring for children and tend to talk to them in the same way. However sometimes midwives retreat behind this form of address as a shield to prevent themselves from having an adult relationship with women. In this way they do not have to reply to questions for which they either do not have the answer, or do not have the authority to answer (Kirkham, 1989). It is important for all women but particularly for the survivor that the midwife is a partner in care and not a wielder of power. For it is the power differential that is the potentially abusive element in the relationship and this is heartening for male midwives to know. For many women who have been abused it is the vulnerability and powerlessness that is so traumatic not the gender of the attendant. There may be some that do not wish to be attended by a man but for many the gender is less relevant than being treated with respect and confidentiality as a decision-making adult.

In the labour ward midwives and obstetricians should sometimes take time out to view the context and procedures as a sexually abused woman might and ask themselves how they can minimize the effects. There is a need to review all the procedures of high tech modern day obstetrics for how many of them have been truly researched and found to be of benefit to the women and their babies? There is growing awareness that many of the procedures are iatrogenic in themselves, for instance, cardiotocography, but they are perpetuated for many reasons not least of all the need for surveillance in all matters to do with women's bodies.

Midwives also need to be aware of the reactions that various women may have which do not necessarily mean that the woman has either a very high or low pain threshold, or is compliant or demanding. Women who make a fuss and need their partners with them at all times may not be overreacting. Most importantly the midwife should be aware of the woman who is dissociating and ask herself why and what she should do to help. (In all likelihood she should keep the woman well and truly focused in the present.)

In the postnatal period midwives are uniquely placed to observe and help women. They know that unusual reactions or obsessive type behaviour may be a sign of impending postnatal depression or difficulties with the mother-infant relationship but they do not always know of the link between these and previous sexual abuse. As the person who cares for her immediately after birth and during the period that the woman is finding her way as a mother, the midwife is ideally placed to spend time with her and to help her explore her feelings. The midwife gives family planning advice and this may act as an opener for the woman to throw out clues about her attitude to the birth and to sex in particular. Anxiety, inadequacy and low self-esteem are precursors of postnatal depression but they are also part of the repertoire of feelings of the sexual abuse survivor and the midwife should be aware of this.

It is important that midwives are sensitive to women and to their needs. This may come about naturally as part of the midwife's personality as well as her education. However, as was discussed earlier, many midwives and perhaps those in particular who are mothers themselves, often confuse their professional caring with their mothering skills. It is possible that a better way of caring could be envisaged if two things were to happen. The first is that midwifery itself is empowered as a profession and develops its own concepts with midwives no longer having to work with one eye looking over their shoulder for their master's permission to speak. The second is that they are provided with training and education in the skills of self-awareness and counselling that may be needed to ensure that they can give non-judgemental empathetic care.

Midwives should be sensitive and empathetic in order to help, but before one can help someone else one must be able to help oneself and it must not be forgotten that midwives and obstetricians are part of society. Many health care professionals will have been abused themselves as children and how they have come to terms with it or not will inevitably affect their ability and approach to the care of a woman who is a sexual abuse survivor. They may also be affected by the syndrome of silence and may not have or feel able to disclose their past to anyone. They may still be suffering the aftermath themselves or they may be less affected. It is difficult to generalize but they may have suffered to an extent that interferes with their professional stance, for instance, they may be unable to make close relationships and so retreat behind a professional protective shell. Or they may find that they have a stronger identification with the mother which may lead to conflicts-by-proxy (Furniss, 1991). This potential cause of personal distress may be a destructive situation for the midwife or obstetrician and will not lead to good care for the mother. The caring professions are notorious for not caring about themselves and it is important that this subject is exposed to the light of day and professionals themselves are given counselling and support in order that they can break the collusion of silence which the perpetrators of abuse so successfully achieve.

CHAPTER TWELVE

Alternative Lifestyles

Sapphic love affairs by no means run counter to the traditional distinction of the sexes; they involve in most cases an acceptance of femininity not its denial.
Simone De Beauvoir, *The Second Sex.*

Sexual practices between people of the same gender have been around a long time but homosexuals have not. Homosexuality as a descriptive term for the person was invented in the 1860s (Weeks, 1991). Before that it was the activity that was an offence or a sin, for example, sodomy carried the death sentence in Britain until 1861. The person was not considered to have a personality problem or defect needing counselling or medical treatment, he was just a person being sinful who needed to be punished. It was thought to be always a 'he' because, as Queen Victoria is reputed to have said, 'ladies would never engage in such despicable acts'. In the years following the 1860s more and more emphasis was put upon the person as being a deviant, invert or pervert. The question of the nature of homosexuality occupied many of the sexologists of the age. Havelock-Ellis, Freud, and Krafft-Ebing busied themselves with the definition of normality and the consideration of homosexuality as natural or pathological condition to be tolerated or cured. Unfortunately, like religion, sexuality is not a realm of human experience that lies outside of politics and its considerations and so homosexuality came under the scrutiny of the lawmakers.

In Britain at the end of the 19th century there were a number of powerful political and social movements that concentrated upon making society vice free. There were many factors involved, not least of which was a fear that the British Empire was in decline and needed strong, healthy stock. In attempting to achieve this the Victorians left a legacy of repression and moralistic attitudes to many aspects of society but particularly in the realm of sexual activity. Sexual activity being as it is so intricately involved with kinship and reproduction was seen to be of public importance not a purely private affair between individuals.

This led to it becoming a matter for medical, social and legal intervention in the name of health care, moral and social rectitude.

Since Victorian times and until the mid-1970s there have been many theories put forward to explain homosexuality in terms of medical and psychological pathology, social deviancy and biological determinism. It has been variously considered a psychological disturbance, which being a sickness could be spotted early in life and a cure attempted (Bayer, 1981), and as a social problem in which the person has deviated from the path of normality due to factors in his or her upbringing, such as a weak father and a dominant mother. (This is a neat theory which kills two birds with one stone, not only does it explain the 'problem' but it covertly signals to women to remain in the role of passive little woman'.) Freud was a notable exception to this thinking for he argued that homosexuals were not exceptions in society and to think of them as such and to separate them off from mankind as a group of special character was wrong (Freud, 1962). Homosexuality has only relatively recently been removed from the list of psychosexual disorders of the Diagnostic and Statistical Manual of Mental and Physical Disorders (3rd edition, 1973) of the American Psychiatric Association. It will take a long while until all vestiges of this are removed from medical thinking because the consideration of it as a pathology is tenacious. (See Kromemeyer (1980) p.7 who considers that the homosexual is an individual who has deeply rooted emotional deprivation and disturbances originating from infancy and whose capacity for true maturation, for healthy growth and love is crippled.)

Male homosexuality, even between consenting adults, has been a criminal offence until relatively recently and even now in 1994 the age of consent has not been brought into line with the rest of the population. Sixteen-year-old boys can have sex with 16- year-old girls, but not with other 16- year-old boys. This anomaly is not so surprising when one considers the homophobic persecution that gay people had and still have to put up with. The 1950s were a particular time of oppression, particularly in the United States, when homosexuality was linked with communism as an Un-American activity which had to be rooted out and punished at all costs. This led to vulnerable people from small towns banding together in areas of big cities, for example, Greenwich Village in New York. As their reputation grew so other homosexuals migrated there and communities were formed. Homosexuals were at one time lumped together with all other sexual minorities as sex offenders but gradually, as the gay rights movement gained members and momentum, they have been spilt off and other categories such as transsexuals, transvestites and sado masochists have been identified as the sex offenders. Regardless of the progress of liberal views with regard to homosexual behaviour there is one aspect of sexuality that is firmly protected by society and that is children's sexuality. In both England and America there are strict laws to protect children's innocence and anyone whose sexuality is not conventional, i.e. heterosexual and married, is suspect.

Adults who deviate too much from conventional standards of sexual conduct are often denied contact with the young, even their own. Custody laws permit the state to steal the children of anyone whose erotic activities appear questionable to a judge presiding over family court matters. (Rubin, 1993)

This fear of being declared an 'unfit' teacher, social worker, health care worker or parent keeps many gay people in the 'closet'. Even gays who come out in the social aspects of their lives may find it very difficult to do so at work or with their family. The old attitudes die hard and there is still an immense amount of prejudice and homophobia in society at large. This may extend to parents who can blame themselves for something they have done wrong in the person's upbringing and can be filled with shame and self-blame.

Just as not every heterosexual is a fit and proper person to convey moral values to the next generation, neither is it true that every homosexual is unfit. Even though the laws on sexual control are very strong there are even stronger social sanctions on people to conform.

This is of particular relevance to lesbians and, contrary to Queen Victoria's assumptions, lesbians do exist. In some ways gay women have been more fortunate than men in that they have not been persecuted in law quite as much, but that is not to say they have not suffered in other ways. They have had their fair share of 'cures' including the once popular clitoridectomy. That lesbians have existed for a very long time is evident by their name, taken as it is from the followers of the seventh century Greek female poet Sappho on the island of Lesbos. Lesbians seem to have a history divided into three periods of time. There is the distant and ill-recorded pre Judeo-Christian past when the Earth Mother Goddess was worshipped in many parts of the world and the fertility and sexuality of women was venerated. This was the time of female power and is attested to by many female carvings dating back to the stone age. It was also a time when 'given that men's role in reproduction was also uncertain, men were probably viewed as superfluous to the health and continuance of the species' (Achterberg, 1990). This period included the time of Sappho who was renowned as a lyric poet and who subjectified rather than objectified women and their sexuality in her poems. This age ended with the rise of Judaism, Christianity and the other patriarchal religions and began a period of decline for women and their power. This continued unabated and culminated in the killing of nine million women in the witch hunts, many of whom are said to have been lesbians (Wolf, 1980). This theory is not universally held and indeed is challenged by writers such as Monique Wittig (1993) who claims that this is 'symmetrical with the biologizing interpretation produced up to now by the class of men'.

Lesbianism remained very unobtrusive until the early part of the 20th century when it became quite fashionable in literary and artistic circles to be bisexual. Notable women were Vita Sackville West and Gertrude Stein. They were able to have such freedom mainly because of their wealth and privileged social positions. This freedom was not extended to the lower social classes who were very restrained by legal, religious and medical mores which variously condemned homosexual practices as unlawful, sinful or sick. Lesbians did, however, form a large part of the early womens' movement, partly because they were not married and had the freedom to be political activists. As women became stronger and demanded the right to be independent of men and have exclusive friendships with other women, they began to be perceived by men as a threat. Part of the answer to this was to 'discover' the sexuality of the married woman which could be awakened only by her husband and to marginalize lesbians to the edges of society as not being real or complete women. Lesbianism was thus to remain relatively obscure and unspoken of until the late 1950s.

Humanistic research from the 1970s onwards has rejected the notion of pathology and considers and presents homosexuality in terms of life choices and alternative lifestyles. Gay men and women are not considered a breed apart, but as men and women who have the right to pursue their right to personal happiness and self fulfilment with as much dignity and freedom as any member of the public. Liberal humanism 'functions to remove lesbianism from the public domain' (Kitzinger, 1987) and leans heavily on the work of Kinsey *et al* (1953) to show that the physiological response is the same in either heterosexual and homosexual acts. It puts forward a model that does not categorize between homosexual and heterosexual but is 'conceptualized as a matter of sexual preference or choice of lifestyles' (Kitzinger, 1987) with the lesbian being seen as capable of mental well-being, a participative and constructive role in society and the pursuance of individual life goals. This assimilative model has been reviewed by Celia Kitzinger (*op. cit.*) who in her critique points out that both homosexuality and

133

heterosexuality are social constructions. In addition, liberal humanistic theory runs contrary to the tenets of radical lesbianism. One of the most obvious differences is that lesbian women are not just like any other women because they are subjected to specific oppression as lesbians and as such must bring the private into the public social arena. There must be lesbian ideas, lesbian identities and lesbian politics.

Lesbian women face prejudice in many aspects of their lives. Religion which is a comfort to many women may be fully denied to lesbians in that it considers homosexuality a sin. This originated with the Israelites, who like all tribes were concerned about matters of kinship and tribal boundaries. What was, perhaps, a necessity at the time for the procreation of children and continuance of the tribe has been taken on board as a prescription for living, and indulgence in sexual acts not designed to procreate children becomes a sin for people to wrestle with mentally. This means that lesbian women act in one of three ways towards their religion; they may leave altogether, they may suffer in silence by not 'coming out' and attend services incognito so to speak, or they may declare themselves and attempt to bring about change.

The social, medical, legal and religious forces come together as one great tidal wave of pressure against lesbian women in the area of motherhood. Lesbians mothers are extremely vulnerable to power dynamics of what Weeks (1981) calls a moral panic. This he says,

crystallises widespread fears and anxieties, and often deals with them not by seeking the real causes of the problems and conditions which they demonstrate but by displacing them on to 'Folk Devils' in an identified social group (often the 'immoral' or 'degenerate').

Children have and always will be the focus of societies hopes and ambitions for the future and as such are a precious resource for the transmission of the culture. This is usually the culture of the dominant ideology which in Western society is patriarchal heterosexuality. Mothers then have a very important role in this transmission and as such must be subjected to careful social surveillance and control. Lesbians who are, or wish to become mothers in a homophobic society pose a threat to this order, and as such can be seen as one of Week's folk devils. They may also be seen by other lesbians in two ways. Negatively, they may be considered to have fallen into the role proscribed for them as woman's biological destiny and an agent of forced production. Or, positively, they may be considered to be accomplishing a woman's most creative act and gaining control of the production of children.

There are two main groups of lesbian women who are mothers. They are those who enter into a conventional heterosexual relationship and may marry. They may or may not be able to identify themselves as lesbian for many years and bear their children within the relationship. They may find that the awareness of their sexuality creeps up on them slowly or they may fall in love with another woman quite suddenly. As they become more and more certain of their sexuality they are left with two courses of action. They may be fearful of the legal and social discrimination that they may have to face, and in particular the possibility of losing their children, and so they sit tight, deny themselves and do nothing. This is obviously a very damaging situation for both the woman and her male partner. To live with someone who cannot share sexual intimacy and emotional fulfilment can be very destructive to one's self-esteem and to the relationship as a whole. It is highly likely that the relationship will break down and divorce will ensue. The woman is still left with the problem of 'coming out' because it is still fraught with difficulties for her. There is still a potential for trauma both to herself, her children, her parents, and her ex-partner. She may be handing over a weapon to wound herself with.

Or she may decide to leave the relationship, get a divorce and live with a female partner within the lesbian community. This, in itself, is a very challenging and frightening concept. At its most challenging, as Wittig (1993) points out, it may mean that identifying oneself as a lesbian means leaving behind the recognized concept of woman itself. She maintains (p.108) that, the designated subject (lesbian) is *not* a woman, either economically, or politically, or ideologically. For what makes a woman is a specific social relation to a man......

.The least of the challenge is the assumption of a new social role and financial status that many divorced women with children find themselves in.

The other main group of women are those who become mothers as confirmed lesbians. They have several options in the manner of becoming pregnant. The woman may choose to have sexual intercourse with a man (a stud) if she feels that she (and her lover) can handle it or she may have artificial insemination by donor (AID). Very often the donor is a gay man who is fully part of the discussion, understands the issues and is willing to establish a friendly but non-proprietal relationship. She may inseminate herself, or her lover may do it for her. She may also choose to visit a clinic and request AID using sperm from a sperm bank. This is not unproblematic because of the social controls which may inhibit her freedom of access.

If the woman is infertile she is faced with another problem. Infertility programmes are not purely medical affairs. In Maseide (1991), Parsons described medical practitioners as agents of social control where both the doctor and the patient are subject to the power of the social system.

Power was not understood as the doctor's power over the patient, but as an general capacity and medium to secure the performance of binding obligations in a social system. (Maseide, 1991)

Women are not autonomous and are not in control of their own fertility in society and this is made very clear with regard to infertile lesbian women who wish to become mothers. The State always exerts authority over the power of reproduction even though as Warnock (1984) affirms there is a commitment to the idea of the "maternal bond, uterine nurturance being a relationship that is thought to combine the moral with the biological". It is concerned with kinship and descent. Descent according to Lewis (1976) (p.236) 'may become a basic principle of social organization on which many vital rights, duties and interests turn'. These matters will become stunningly obvious to a lesbian who wishes to be considered for infertility treatment. She will have to jump through many a hoop to prove her fitness to become a mother and to have use of the resources of the State. It may also become obvious that doctors do not work in a value free setting dealing purely with the anatomical and physiological issues.

On becoming pregnant the lesbian will find herself as a recipient of maternity care. This involves a type of institutional prejudice which is so covert that its members are probably unaware of it at a personal level and cannot be objectively defined (Kitzinger, 1987). However, for lesbians, like other marginalized groups, who suffer from the effects of discrimination, it is part of their reality. For example, their invisibility alone may be considered prejudicial. This invisibility is similar to the colour blindness experienced by black people within the service. The refusal to acknowledge that a pregnant lesbian group exists and is in any way different from other pregnant women is actually a liberal homophobic attitude which is,

in fact a profoundly homosexual view in that it represents the liberal refusal to notice and attempt to dissolve the specificities of homosexual existence, and contributes to the 'dehomosexualizing' of homosexuals. (Dannecker, 1981)

All through the pregnancy and birth a lesbian will be treated as if she is heterosexual, for example, there may be visiting restrictions where only husbands or fathers are allowed in at certain times. Her female partner may not be acknowledged as the other parent, or if it is recognized that she is in a lesbian relationship the full force of the social and health care services will in all likelihood come into play.

The biggest threat to lesbian mothers is that of having their children taken away from them. The fear engendered is not groundless because it continues to happen, as a judgement as recently as September 1993 confirms. Sharon Bottoms lost the custody of her son Tyler to her disapproving mother (Tisdall, 1993). The judge agreed with the grandmother that the child might grow up unable to tell the difference between men and women if he remained with his mother and her live-in lesbian lover.

As soon as a pregnant woman is identified as a lesbian, concerns will be raised about her fitness for parenthood. This may be covert and again it may not. Her lifestyle will come under scrutiny for the baby's sake. Society's fear is that the child will not have appropriate role models of either sex and will grow up sexually confused. There is no evidence so far that this is indeed the case and the lesbian point of view is that the child will be allowed to grow and develop within a non-sexist culture which can only be beneficial. It is necessary that professionals involved in this area of work have enough self-awareness to ensure that they always act objectively and without prejudice. As society becomes more open and less restrictive, the consequences of such scrutiny may not be quite as devastating for the lesbian mother as it once might have been, but nevertheless there is still necessity for caution.

Lesbian mothers may have a great deal of support from within the community but not necessarily so. This is because there is not a single lesbian identity and just as one woman may consider motherhood essential for her and her partner's fulfilment, so another lesbian may consider that having children is contrary to the ideology of the released woman. Or yet again it might be considered that bearing children is acceptable as long as there is escape from the confines of a constricting family unit and children are brought up in a communal family. Generally though, they are well supported and there are very often women's groups, lesbian associations and local self-help groups who will give them help, legal advice and support in their effort to keep and protect their child.

Older children, particularly teenagers, may have difficulty in coming to terms with their mother's (or father's) homosexuality. Adolescence is a time of stress and strain in the development of one's sexual identity and the burden of having to deal with a parent's revelations may be too much for the teenager to cope with. It may mean that they opt to stay with the father and not get involved. They may feel ashamed and threatened and have difficulty in expressing their anxieties. This can make the lesbian mother feel bereft, distressed and full of grief and loss. Boys, in particular, may feel that they are being rejected because of their maleness. There are, however, teenagers who do not react like this, and whilst they do have to make adjustments, are quite able to cope and are supportive of their mothers whilst being secure in their own sexuality. There always seems to be a fear that children brought up by homosexuals will be homosexual themselves, but this is not a causal relationship. As homosexuals will point out they themselves were brought up by heterosexuals without becoming heterosexual. Most lesbian women want only that their children grow up to be in a satisfactory, liberated and fulfilling emotional relationship.

It may be that the woman decides that it is in her children's best interests if she gives them up, but if she does she will find herself in a catch 22 situation, for she may be stigmatized as selfish and an unnatural mother for choosing a lover before her children. If she does not there are issues to be faced with having her children live with her. The main problems are similar to those experienced with any new partner, i.e. trying to balance the love and attention that she gives to both parties and ensuring equity for all and trying to play down jealousies. Some women hide the relationship from the children and others are quite open. It is all a matter of individual choice.

The options for people who want to have children, such as adoption and fostering are also problematic for homosexuals and until very recently it has been almost impossible. There are lobby groups such as Stonewall in England that are pressurizing to eradicate prejudice against gays and lesbians who wish to foster. They have recently been successful in the case of a lesbian couple in a long-term relationship who have won their three year battle to become foster parents (Weale, 1993). Whether this is a breakthrough or not remains to be seen because the junior health minister Tim Yeo made it quite clear that in most cases a child was better placed with a 'mum and dad', and the Government expected local authorities to make every effort to achieve this. One of the statements made in this case was that they were able to offer a lot in a 'very calm, loving, ordinary household'. This, coupled with the result goes some way towards confirming Rubin's (1993) hypothesis that there is a line of demarcation between acceptable and non-acceptable behaviour and although most homosexuality is still on the wrong side of the line, some forms such as long-term monogamous relationships are inching towards the border. As Rubin (*op. cit.*) also says it correlates with the ideologies of racism in which the dominant group are granted virtue. It also denies variety in matters sexual whereas in every other walk of life variety is almost a necessity.

Two varieties that are possibly of relevance to a discussion of sexuality and motherhood are those of transvestitism and transsexualism. Both are in the main male phenomena and say a lot about gender issues and the construction of the feminine and masculine roles. Transvestites are very much men. They may dress as women, but to them the penis is of major importance. Not only do they want to keep it but they revel in its capacity for erection, particularly when arrayed as a female. As Stoller (1968) points out, transvestitism is the way such a man has of handling strong feminine identification without feeling that his masculinity is being submerged by feminine wishes. He gets a kick out of it and sexual excitement from knowing that under his most feminine of clothes there is still a functioning penis. In no way do transvestites want to become women. In whatever flimsy underwear they dress, they still want reassurance of their potency, ideally by having a large erect penis. These men statistically tend to be middle-class, heterosexual and married, and what is more they stay married. For whatever reason their wives tend, after a while, to accept their play acting and join in by helping them to choose clothes and makeup, and by calling them by their feminine name when they are cross-dressed. One interesting aspect of transvestitism is the way that these men take on board the rigid, narrow stereotype of femininity. Not for them the leggings and t-shirt, it has to be the basque and the chiffon nightie at the very least. Stoller suggests that there is no such person as a transvestite woman, only transsexual women because it is rare for a woman to become sexually excited merely by the wearing of male attire. Feminist issues, women's problems, women's rights and motherhood are of no interest to them as transvestites, although they may be of interest to them from a man's perspective in their everyday lives.

Transsexuals highlight a more interesting and complicated set of issues from a woman's point of view. They (the majority are male) have the problem of feeling that they are a female trapped in a male body. The initial problem seems to result from the powerful effect that society has on people to ensure that they conform to the prescribed gender role and its ascribed behavioural characteristics. As these males cannot or will not live up to the cultural norm for men they identify with the opposite sex, or to be more precise their interpretation of what the opposite sex is and feels like. This, as in the case of the transvestites, is usually a very stereotypical view of women and transsexuals both before and after surgery are often admired for their beauty, long eyelashes and softly feminine clothes. They also stereotypically associate maleness with the presence of a penis and scrotum and so, unlike the transvestite who glories in his penis and the sexual excitement he gains from it, the transsexual's penis causes him nothing but despair.

It is possibly true to say that the transsexual as we know him is a product of and can only exist in a male dominated patriarchal society. Whatever the reason for their existence, there has arisen a whole team of medical professionals to enable their transition to womanhood. John Money at the John Hopkins Hospital in America originally started the work by specializing in the correction of hermaphroditism and as Sally Vincent (1993) put it, he extended the courtesy to 'anyone else who fails to comply with the standards of sexual normality'. So transsexuals, who first must live the stereotype, i.e. they can have hormonal treatment and develop breasts and live as women for a fixed term, usually three years or so, can then have their genitalia reassigned - their penis and testicles cut off. A space is scooped out of the perineum and highly sensitive skin from the scrotum is used to line a newly fashioned `vagina'. With this and the aid of a multiplicity of procedures such as electrolysis of the beard, removal of the Adam's apple and shortening of the legs, the transsexual is now corrected of his gender dysphoria and is now a woman. Or is he? That is the conundrum. For what is a woman?

The transsexual is as Raymond (1979) points out,

> unfolding a world view of patriarchy that explains its origins, beliefs and practices. Transsexuals are living out two basic patriarchal myths: single parenthood by the father (male mothering) and the making of women according to man's image. Both myths are writ large in all the religions of manmade civilization.

Now the problem is one of nature versus nurture. Is he a woman or is he a medicalized man without a penis and scrotum, a eunuch in fact. This is the intellectual problem that faces anyone considering these issues. It could be said that he cannot be a woman on two counts. He is biologically not a product of nature for he does not posses the XX chromosomes and the internal reproductive organs. Neither is he a product of nurture for he has been socialized as a male, even though he thought he was a woman trapped in male body it was an internal idea rather than an everyday reality as it is for woman who have been so from birth. One feminist point of view is that he is a eunuch and like the eunuchs of old is capable of wielding great power. One way of doing so is to invade and penetrate women not with his penis but with his whole being. He invades and penetrates women's space in a very profound way and so is typically masculine. He is also free of the biological vulnerability of women, their ability to reproduce, and so is free to pursue career choices in a very masculine way. He is, in fact, no more a woman than before. This obsession with the removal of the penis also serves to highlight the significance of the penis as a symbol of maleness.

There is another view that can be explored with regard to transsexuals. If as Monica Wittig (1993) considers there is no such thing as men and women but merely social constructions, and what makes a woman is 'a specific social relationship to a man, a relationship that we have previously called servitude', then surely a physically constructed woman can also be socially constructed. Or can she? Can she and should she be allowed to get married and adopt children? Can she really be a feminist? Can she be a lesbian?

As a final postscript there are two things to say, first there is no evidence that the majority of transsexuals achieve their goal of happiness following surgery. Secondly, little has been said about the plight of female to male transsexuals because even though the surgical work has been on-going from the 1950s, there has been little in the way of development of expertise in the manufacture of the penis for such women. Is this because it is too precious an organ to give to a woman?

CHAPTER THIRTEEN

Sexual Health

> *The one facet of the AIDS epidemic that I think almost everyone prefers to*
> *overlook is this:*
> *Something infectious is going around.*
> Larry Kramer (1990)

Ten years ago student midwives were being taught that women were protected from the HIV virus through heterosexual intercourse because the ph of the vagina was acid. Likewise it was part of the myth that lesbian loving did not carry any risk. We now know both to be untrue. It was killing women while these statements were being made. It was killing women before we knew it existed and it will go on killing women until it is defeated. The literature until quite recently concentrated on HIV-related illness as a mainly man's disease but although it is known that the first recorded case was an English seaman in 1959, it is not as well known that the first recorded female deaths were those of a Norwegian sailor's wife and daughter in 1976 (Froland *et al*, 1988) . This is not to say that these people were the first to become infected but rather that they were the first to be positively identified (Mercey, Bewley and Brocklehurst, 1993). Women are very much at risk from HIV and AIDS and in some parts of the world it has become the leading cause of death among women of reproductive age. HIV infection awareness serves to highlight the health risks and issues surrounding the sexuality of women which are considerable, particularly for the poor and the underprivileged.

Many people are oblivious of the HIV virus, they either do not know what it is or what its effect can be on their own lives, or they do not want to know. They are walking through a holocaust with their eyes shut. But not thinking about it will not make it go away. HIV is here and it will not avoid an unthinking person, just as it does not avoid any man or woman rich or poor, because it cannot, it has no power of discrimination. HIV is simply a virus, the human immunodeficiency virus.

It is a lymphotropic virus consisting of ribonucleic acid (RNA) which enters a host cell and as it multiplies a reverse enzyme acts to transform it into deoxyribonucleic acid (DNA). This is the opposite from the usual happening of RNA being formed from DNA and so the virus is termed a retrovirus. Like all viruses HIV is capable of subtle changes and this is becoming evident by the presence of other forms such as the recently named HIV 2 which has been found in West Africa. This is related to HIV 1 but is substantially different, even though it causes similar illnesses.

Originally the virus was isolated in France and because it came from a patient with enlarged lymph glands it was called lymphadenopathy associated virus or LAV. Meanwhile in America it was isolated from AIDS patients and named human T lymphotropic virus Type III (HTLV-III). Nowadays it is common practice to name it after its effect on the immune system, human immunodeficiency virus.

Resistance to infection comes about by the action of specialized cells throughout the body, but which are mainly found in the blood, the spleen and the lymph nodes. One particular type, the T lymphocytes, attack other cells which are colonized by viruses and induce a sensitivity reaction. A sub-group of these, the T4 cells or T-helper cells, promote the response, whilst another group, the T8 or T-suppressor cells, dampen the response down. The virus attacks the T4 cells directly by attaching itself to a receptor on their surface the CD4 antigen. It enters and replicates itself by changing the genetic structure and making it a virtual virus factory. The immune system swings into action to make antibodies to the virus but they seem to be incapable of actually eliminating the virus. Meanwhile the T-suppressor cells begin to dampen down the immunocellular activity. T4 cells are destroyed and lost from the body. The ratio is then completely reversed, and whereas previously T4 cells outnumbered T8 by two to one the opposite is now true with T8 cells being double that of T4 cells. Macrophages also have the CD4 antigen and so the HIV is also able to gain entry to them. The macrophages are not destroyed by the HIV but become an important reservoir for their multiplication. HIV has also been isolated from neural tissue (and it a possible cause of dementia). The overall effect is a reduction in the body's capacity to fight disease and the body is then at risk from any opportunistic infection that it comes into contact with.

Once in the bloodstream, HIV can be transported to all parts of the body. It has been found in all the systems of the body, the gastrointestinal, the skeletal, the reproductive, and the nervous. It has been particularly found in high concentrations in semen and in fact seems to reproduce very easily in the sperm cells. It is also found in cervical and vaginal mucous, the endometrium and in the placenta. Although it can be found in all the systems it does not seem to be of high concentration in saliva, but blood, semen and vaginal mucous are thought to be the major means of transmission, and of course, the higher the concentration the more transmissible is the virus from the infected person.

HIV does not usually cause symptoms immediately. It is a slow acting virus and 'current progression to AIDS after an initial HIV infection seems to be 50 per cent at ten years" (Richardson, 1989) . It was thought until quite recently that women progressed to AIDS more quickly than men following the initial exposure to the virus but this is now thought to be incorrect, rather, it is thought that women are less likely to be diagnosed as HIV positive as quickly as men. Following an AIDS diagnosis the mean survival rate is approximately two years. Some people who are HIV positive do have symptoms but do not have AIDS. The virus can cause a range of symptoms of which the acquired immune deficiency syndrome (AIDS) is the worst. The most mild is a persistent swelling of the lymph nodes termed persistent generalized lymphadenopathy (PGL). People with more serious symptoms may not have the opportunistic infections and cancers associated with AIDS and have what is defined as ARC or AIDS-related complex (Reeler, 1990). The most serious progression is to AIDS itself where the body's immune system is seriously damaged and the person is susceptible to a syndrome or group of illnesses such as rare cancers, for example Kaposi's sarcoma (KS), and often fatal infections such as uncommon pneumocystis carinii pneumonia (PCP).

HIV is a very fragile virus and cannot survive for long outside the body. It is not possible to acquire the infection by sitting near somebody, by drinking out of the same cup or swimming in the same pool. The virus is not transmitted by droplet, through the air or by mosquitos. It is transmitted through sexual intercourse either vaginally or anally and in some cases orally if blood, semen or vaginal secretions from an infected person is allowed to enter the body. It can also be transmitted via contaminated blood products usually by sharing needles and syringes and particularly if pumping of blood up into the syringe is practised in order to get every bit of the drug into the body. Unsterilized needles, syringes and other equipment may also be used either by formal or informal health care workers in many parts of the world and are known to be a cause of transmission (Merson, 1990). Sometimes it is communicated by the infusion of unscreened and/or untreated blood products, which is now very rare in the developed countries but is still a reality in less developed parts of the world.

Children can be affected by vertical transmission in utero across the placenta, at birth or in the postnatal period through breastmilk from an infected mother. Women inseminated by artificial means may be at risk if semen from an infected donor is used. This is highly unlikely if semen from a sperm bank is used because the donor will have been screened but it is a risk that women who self-inseminate run unless they are absolutely sure that the donor is uninfected.

Initially HIV and AIDs were associated with gay men and promiscuity which not only was incorrect but left 'the moral majority' feeling unjustifiably safe. For not only is the virus indiscriminate in its choice of host, it is as easy to catch by heterosexual as it is by homosexual contact and it cannot differentiate the virgin from the prostitute. Unfortunately it is easy for sections of the population to assume a moral stance and compare it with a plague from heaven for people's perceived misdemeanours. This type of thinking also encourages the development of the concept of risk groups and so people who do not identify themselves with these groups can consider themselves safe. Sadly, this is the biggest misconception of all, for there are no risk groups only risk behaviours. Neither promiscuity nor monogamy guarantee or protect from HIV infection. HIV infection is contracted when infected body fluids enter the body of an uninfected person. It is that simple.

Much of the literature with regard to the signs and symptoms of HIV infection have concentrated on the manifestations in men. This is quite reasonable as the majority of sufferers in most parts of the developed world have indeed been men. However more and more it is being recognized that great numbers of women in the undeveloped parts of the world and increasingly in the West are suffering from the infection. There are probably quite marked differences in the way the infection presents in women from the way it does in men, just as there is in most sexually transmitted diseases, but as yet there has been very little research to confirm this (New Jersey Women and AIDS Network, 1990). Affecting as it does the reproductive tract it results in menstrual symptoms and irregularities which are obviously unique to women and Kaposi's sarcoma does not seem to affect women (Reeler, 1990).

About two to eight weeks after contact approximately ten per cent of people will present with an acute infection, the first symptoms of which are usually a sore throat, swollen glands, aches and pains reminiscent of influenza and perhaps a skin rash. The remainder of the infected population are asymptomatic and although antibodies to HIV are produced they may remain like this for many years before developing symptoms. Under the communicable diseases classification (CDC) this is termed stage I. The person may remain asymptomatic or have a subclinical deterioration in immune function which is stage II. The symptoms of the acute infection usually last slightly longer than normal but do disappear except for the swollen glands which may persist and become a progressive generalized lymphadenopathy which is stage III of the condition. Most people do not associate these symptoms with the possibility of HIV infection. Women may also experience changes in their menstrual pattern and some have loss of, or mid-cycle bleeding and a lowering of fertility.

As the HIV multiplies in the body the more likely the person is to develop symptoms and go on to stage IV. At first these may be mild and include a general feeling of malaise and tiredness with muscle and joint pains and loss of weight. There are very often fevers particularly with drenching night sweats and pruritus and skin rashes. One of the most common infections is candida albicans (thrush) which presents as white, curd-like plaques on the inside of the vagina or on the glans penis or anal area and is accompanied by a highly irritating white discharge. It may also present in the mouth or further down the gastrointestinal tract. Another common infection is herpes zoster or shingles. The early appearance of herpes zoster, oral candida albicans, hairy leucoplakia and constitutional symptoms are considered markers for a poor prognosis. Other problems are genital herpes simplex infections, genital ulcers and genital warts from the human papilloma virus. In women there are conflicting reports regarding pelvic inflammatory disease. Some studies (Carpenter, 1991) have found that it is a cause of more frequent and severe pelvic inflammatory disease whilst others (Byrne et al, 1989) have not found it to be a significant factor. Abnormal cervical cells and cervical epithelial neoplasia have been found to occur at a younger age in HIV positive women (Nelson et al, 1991) and if untreated progress through all the stages of cervical cancer through to invasive carcinoma more quickly in HIV positive women (Berer and Ray, 1993). Other major conditions which usually indicate serious immunodeficiency and impending death are oral candida particularly oesophageal thrush and pneumocystis carinii pneumonia (PCP) which is usually very rare as it is only passed on if the recipient is also immunodeficient (CDR, 1994). The majority of people with AIDS develop PCP at some stage and it is the most common cause of death in American women with AIDS. Tuberculosis, brain cell damage due to meningitis, cytomegalovirus or toxoplasmosis, chronic diarrhoea, cancers of the skin and lymphatic system, arthritis and heart disease are also either singly, but usually in combination, responsible for the death of AIDS victims.

HIV infections in women are on the increase and AIDS has become a leading cause of death in women of reproductive age in major cities in the Americas, Western Europe and Sub Saharan Africa (*op. cit.*). This is not the case as yet in the United Kingdom, although there have been 2910 women infected with HIV-1 in the ten years from 1984 to 1994 (CDR, 1994) and 387 deaths from AIDS from January 1982 until March 1994. To date there have been 676 pregnancies in 520 HIV infected women and since 1989 the pregnancy rate is averaging at 104 per year (Newell and Peckham, 1993). This being so it is worth considering the effect of HIV on the pregnancy and vice versa.

HIV infection does not seem to have a major effect on the outcome of pregnancy per se (Richardson, 1989). There is no excess of fetal loss or other problems such as growth retardation, congenital abnormalities or prematurity. Although these do occur they are more closely associated with other risk factors such as socio-economic influences, drug abuse and smoking. Likewise the effect of pregnancy on HIV infection is not major. There is a slow and steady decline in T4 cell count but in studies with matched pregnant and non pregnant controls the decline is similar (Richardson, 1989). The problem with this is that the numbers involved were very small and it is difficult to be definite about the validity in extrapolation to the wider population. Likewise the studies that have involved women with severe immune deficiency have been limited and the findings inconclusive. Since the early signs and symptoms of the disease, e.g. tiredness, are very similar to those of pregnancy itself, there may be delay in diagnosing and treating complications of HIV infection. Some authors (Mercey, Bewley and Brocklehurst, 1993) maintain that this is an important indication for screening in pregnancy.

It is extremely difficult and time-consuming to screen for the virus itself so antibody tests have proven to be a relatively simple way of detecting the presence of HIV. When a person has become infected with the virus, antibodies are formed which, whilst reducing the damage to the immune system for a number of years, do not actually destroy the virus itself. The antibodies are usually detected in the blood about six weeks after infection. The period before the antibodies are produced is known as a window and even during this time the person is actually infected and infectious. After a positive HIV antibody test most people are offered a thorough investigation and examination to look for clinical evidence of the infection. This includes a full blood count because anaemia, lymphopoenia, neutropoenia and thrombocytopoenia may occur. T4 cell counts are very useful but there are diurnal fluctuations and so they must be assessed at the same time of the day. Above 500 X $10^6/l$ major opportunistic infections are unlikely but as they fall so more and more infections are likely with pneumocystis carinii appearing when the T4 cells have fallen to about 100 X $10^6/l$ or less. P24 antigenaemia occurs at seroconversion and with a low T4 cell count is indicative of the imminence of symptoms. On examination there may be any one or more of the following signs and symptoms: raised temperature, weight loss, anaemia, retinitis, hepatomegaly, splenomegaly, lymphadenopathy, herpes zoster, warts, and respiratory problems. There may be diarrhoea, abdominal pain, headaches, coughs, colds, and night sweats.

Sexual intercourse between men still remains the largest exposure category among HIV-1 infections accounting for 60 per cent of the cumulative total of the past ten years in the UK. Infection in women is to date approximately ten per cent that of men, and of those the majority have probably acquired the virus either from a high risk partner or from a partner abroad, or they are an injecting drug user. A woman may be infected before or during pregnancy and both will cause her to face dilemmas and make decisions about whether to have a baby or not. It has been said earlier that there is a lowering of fertility in the woman who is HIV positive. This may indeed be true or it may be that HIV positive women practice safe sex and their partners wear a condom. Or it may be that they are following the advice of health professionals such as the American College of Obstetrics and Gynaecology (ACOG) which in 1987 recommended that infected persons should be discouraged from becoming pregnant and should be offered help with family planning (Berer and Ray, 1993). By 1990 this advice had been modified to urge that professionals respect women's choices regardless of her reproductive status. This was because it is more and more recognized that people have the right to an informed choice. Many women will take the risk that their baby will be among the 60-85 per cent of children who are born without the infection. It is sometimes very difficult for a healthy woman to face both her own and her baby's mortality and it may be that she cannot believe in the imminence of death. For others it may be that in reality they do not have the choice to avoid pregnancy. This is very true in some cultures where there is a high infant mortality rate and a women's reproductive capacity does not truly belong to herself but to her husband and his family. It may also be that evading pregnancy is not a possibility because that would mean informing the partner of the HIV status and facing divorce, social ostracism or physical maltreatment.

Achieving pregnancy is not without its dangers and difficulties. An HIV positive woman presents a danger to an uninfected partner. It is better if they practice artificial insemination, i.e. they use a condom all of the time but when the woman is ovulating they use a syringe to introduce the semen into her vagina. A condom should be used throughout pregnancy. It is important that if donor sperm is used the HIV status of the donor must be known. If the woman is HIV negative and her partner is positive artificial insemination by an uninfected donor is a far safer option.

It may be that a woman does not know her HIV status before becoming pregnant or she may sero convert during the pregnancy. On finding she is HIV positive she may need to make a decision as to the continuance of the pregnancy or not. She may also find difficulties with the availability of abortion. She may live in a country where it is illegal or difficult to obtain or she herself may have religious or ethical objections. Whether she obtains an abortion or not she will find that she is likely to experience conflicting emotions. She may indeed face hostility and pressure from family or professionals and may submit to having a termination against her will (Ballantyne, 1988). If she decides to have an abortion she may find that there is discrimination against her by the health professionals concerned because there is still lack of knowledge and fear even amongst people who should be more informed than the general public.

If the woman continues with the pregnancy she faces a stressful time not least of which is due to the prospect of her child being infected. As all babies are born HIV positive it is likely to be at least 18 months before she will know for certain one way or another. There is evidence to suppose that the virus can cross the placental barrier and the risk has been variously estimated at 15-20 per cent (Newell and Peckham, 1993) and 25-40 per cent (Richardson, 1989) and is at its greatest in relation to the length of time the woman has been infected and to the presence of symptoms. It is not possible to test the fetus antenatally, for example, with examination of the liquor because the presence of the virus or antibodies may well be the mother's rather than the fetus' own. There is an increased risk of transmission during premature labour and so all positive women need particular advice in pregnancy on how to recognize the signs of early labour. In premature labour they should go to the hospital as early as possible. However the value of tocolytic treatment to prevent premature labour and reduce transmission is still uncertain (Mercey, Bewley and Brocklehurst, 1993).

The aim of care in labour of all women is to provide them with as safe and satisfying an experience as possible with as little trauma as possible. The care of women with HIV or AIDS is no different in this respect. It is, however, extremely important that any invasive procedures are very carefully considered and avoided as far as possible. In order to reduce the risk to the fetus the membranes should not be artificially ruptured, vaginal examinations should be kept to a minimum, and fetal scalp electrodes and fetal blood sampling should be avoided. The labour itself should be treated as normally as possible and there are no contraindications to analgesia. At delivery the aim of the management is to have as normal a delivery as possible with intervention kept to a minimum. It is useful if this is attended by an experienced midwife because, ideally, there should be an intact perineum and episiotomy, forceps and ventouse extraction avoided as much as possible. This is to avoid the risk of transmission to the baby at delivery. It may be that the obstetrician after discussion with the mother decides upon an elective caesarean section. This is particularly so in the event of a twin pregnancy where it is more likely that the first twin is infected. The evidence for the protective effect is not conclusive on this, but some obstetricians believe that there is a lower incidence of vertical transmission in babies born by caesarean section (European Collaborative Study, 1992). There is no evidence to support any deviations from the normal management of the third stage of labour. The baby should be bathed as quickly as is reasonable for his or her condition to remove any maternal blood.

The mother and baby do not need to be isolated in the postnatal period. It is an anxious time anyway for an HIV woman and so to be kept apart from other mothers merely adds to the stress. She should be taught to look after herself and her baby as much as possible and taught how to avoid and or deal with blood leakage and splashes. This woman needs the best and most tender care that a midwife can give and she should be assured confidentiality at all times. The woman herself must decide who she wishes to know and this extends to her family and to her partner. Women should also be offered contraceptive advice and counselling by a trained person following delivery. She will have decisions about her own health, her baby's future care and whether or not to conceive again.

Breastfeeding is highly beneficial to babies and unless there is strong evidence that it is harmful, i.e. the baby can be infected through breast milk as distinct from an infection at or before birth, then it should be recommended. There is very little evidence to date to suggest that breastfeeding by HIV positive mothers who were HIV negative at delivery is harmful except for one study (European Collaborative Study, 1992) where the numbers of breastfeeders to bottlefeeders were so disproportionate that the results were problematic and this is illustrated in a case study in the work of Zeigler *et al*, (1985). Where the mother was HIV positive in pregnancy it may be that the maternal HIV antibodies passed across in the breast milk may have a protective effect upon the infant and there is evidence to support the view that babies infected with HIV at birth develop AIDS more slowly if breastfed than babies who are not (Tozzi *et al*, 1990). It is a very unclear and thorny problem and so, because there may be some risk however small, obstetricians are advising HIV positive women not to breastfeed (Mercey, Bewley and Brocklehurst, 1993) and this is supported by the May 1992 WHO/UNICEF statement (1992). However it is extremely important that women in countries where there is a high infant mortality rate and inadequate supplies of clean water are encouraged to breastfeed whatever their HIV status. HIV infected milk may hypothetically be a risk factor but contaminated or dilute breastmilk substitute is most definitely a killer.

Women (and men) with AIDS or who are HIV positive face discrimination overreaction and outright hostility from many parts of the population and sadly from some health professionals. This is usually based on fear and ignorance which is inexcusable amongst professionals who have a duty to care and to control infection. The control of infection is a two-way process. The midwife or other health care professional must protect herself and other women and babies from infection and must be careful not to introduce infection to the HIV positive women whose immune system is not optimum. Most hospitals and Trusts have infection control policies which, if adhered to, will reduce the risk on both these counts. Initially there was a space suit approach to the problem which it is now acknowledged as unnecessary. There needs to be a common policy which assumes that HIV or hepatitis B may be a possible risk in every case and so staff should avoid being exposed to body fluids. This means wearing gloves when coming into contact with blood, amniotic fluid or vaginal secretions. Needles and sharps must be disposed of in rigid containers and needles must not be resheathed. Protective clothing, glasses, and plastic aprons or water repellent gowns must be worn at delivery. Abrasions on the skin must be covered and gloves worn if necessary until healing has taken place. Any blood splashes must be cleaned up immediately with disinfectant.

All sanitary pads and rubbish must be disposed of correctly (usually in plastic bags).

After delivery the baby should not be aspirated unless absolutely necessary and if so a mouth mucous extractor should only be used if absolutely necessary and then it should be of the type with a protective membrane to prevent aspirate from being drawn up into the midwife's mouth. Babies should be carefully washed, particularly their heads and ears where congealed blood tends to stick, and the midwife should be gloved and wear a plastic apron whilst doing so. The placenta should never be touched whilst ungloved. If blood samples are necessary they should be taken carefully whilst wearing gloves and self-sealing syringe cum bottles used. If it is known that the women is HIV positive then specimens should be labelled with a biohazard label. All non-disposable equipment, e.g. incubators, should be cleaned with an appropriate cleanser such as one per cent sodium hypochlorite solution or two per cent glutaraledehyde, and washed with hot water and detergent, however, wherever possible disposable equipment should be used. When examining the perineum or a caesarean section wound the midwife must wear disposable gloves. General measures should be taken to prevent cross-infection at all times. These include careful hand washing, reduction of traumatic and invasive procedures, careful wound dressing, good aseptic techniques, use of disposable equipment, screening of staff for infection, encouragement of good hygiene and discouragement of visitors with illnesses. If a member of staff suffers a needle stick injury or other cut in contact with blood or body fluid it should be encouraged to bleed by squeezing it and then it should be held under running water. Likewise any blood splashes in the eye, mouth or skin should be well irrigated. There is usually an appropriate accident reporting and follow-up procedure to be followed. Typically it means the injury should be reported on an accident form to the control of infection officer and to the occupational health department and in the case of needle stick injuries a sample of blood is taken and the member of staff is given follow up care by a consultant. The person may also be at risk from Hepatitis B or C. Before an HIV antibody test is performed she or he should be offered counselling.

It is helpful if an HIV positive woman can be seen by the paediatrician before her baby is born because she needs to have as much information as possible and the baby needs to be carefully followed up. It is heartening to know that the transmission rate is less than 50 per cent and could be as low as 15 per cent. At birth most babies are HIV antibody positive due to the presence of maternal antibodies and these may not disappear in an uninfected baby until it is 18 months old. The baby is examined at birth for congenital abnormalities, and signs of drug withdrawal symptoms if its mother is drug user. Investigations will be undertaken for the presence of the virus, cytomegalovirus immune status and a full blood count will be performed. The baby will be followed up at six weeks, 12 weeks and every three months afterwards. There have been no contraindications to immunisations to date and the current advice is that the child should be given all the routine vaccinations except polio which should be given as the killed virus to protect other members of the family who may be immunodeficient. BCG should be given unless the baby is definitely known to be infected. In addition the baby may need to be given vaccinations against influenza and hepatitis B.

If he or she loses antibodies and has no symptoms, this is confirmed at the second visit and the child is declared uninfected and prophylactic treatment e.g. trimethoprim-sulphamethoxazole (septrin) is then stopped. If the baby is infected the earliest infection to appear is pneumocystis carinii pneumonia at about three to six months followed by thrombocytopoenia, candida albicans infections, HIV encephalopathy and bacterial infections. The parents need a great deal of emotional support and advice at this time from healthcare professionals. Families with HIV infected children have been subject to social ostracism in the past and they must be assured that confidentiality is maintained with as few professionals as possible knowing. They must also be educated about the transmission of the virus in order to protect their child and others. So far there have been no reports of transmission between children at play groups or schools.

To date HIV infection in the majority of children and in adults seems to lead to the development of AIDS. There is a small minority of adults who have not developed symptoms as yet. It may be that they never do so but it also may be that the virus has a very long asymptomatic period in some people and they become ill some time in the near future. Treatment is usually directed at the symptoms, e.g. pneumonia. Zidovudine, i.e. 3 azido-3 deoxythymidine (AZT) was initially hailed as a wonder drug for the inhibition of the viral reverse transcriptase activity (Albouker and Swart, 1993). It does seem to be associated with prolongation of adult survival rates in the short-term but has no effect in the long-term. It can cause nausea, vomiting and diarrhoea but seems to have no toxic effects in pregnancy. It will continue to be prescribed for its beneficial effects until a more effective drug is found.

As there is no cure for AIDS the best that can be done is to prevent it and this can be achieved in part by the practice of safe sex. This may not be as easy for women as it sounds. There are two vital components necessary for the reduction in transmission of the HIV virus and they are knowledge and empowerment. Women (and men) need to have the facts about risk reduction and they must also be able to say no to unprotected sex.

Sexual practices can be broken down into three categories, safe, risky and high risk. The practices that come into the safe category are those that do not involve the possibility of blood or semen entering another person's body. These include kissing, cuddling, massage, masturbation either alone or mutual (as long as there are no open cuts on the hands), hugging, body rubbing, non-genital body kissing and acting out fantasies. The use of a vibrator is safe, as long as it is not shared with someone else. Some people will find that they can have a satisfying relationship without needing anything more than this however others will want more.

Behaviour which carries possible risks include oral sex. This is risky to the woman if she takes the penis into her mouth and there is a reproductive tract infection or she allows semen to be emitted into her mouth. Men receiving fellatio seem to be at little risk. For a man it is particularly risky to perform cunnilingus if the woman is having a period or she has a reproductive tract infection. As with fellatio there seems to be little risk to the woman receiving cunnilingus. Contact with the anus either orally (rimming) or with the unprotected fingers or fist is potentially hazardous as is water sports (urinating on each other). Very high risk behaviour involves penetrative vaginal or anal sex without the use of a condom and any practice that causes trauma and bleeding followed by unprotected sex.

There are straightforward methods of reducing the risks and these include some of the following: good personal hygiene for both sexes and men should ensure that the area under the foreskin is clean. A fresh condom should be used on each occasion of sexual intercourse and it should be put on correctly before any contact, i.e. it should not be damaged or torn by hasty unwrapping, the closed end should be squeezed to expel the air, it should be put on the erect penis so it unrolls downwards and it should be held at the base afterwards so it does not slip off the softening penis and spill semen into the vagina. Ideally it should be used in conjunction with a water-based lubricant containing the spermicide nonoxynol-9. The lubricant also makes it less liable to tear. The female condom, the femidon, can also be used and may be more acceptable because the woman can insert it herself before sexual activity starts. Oral sex can be made less risky by the use a condom on the penis or a femidon or diaphragm. Gloves should be used if fingers or hands are going to be inserted into the vagina or anus. Reducing the number of partners also reduces risk in conjunction with the above.

Less straightforward risk reduction involves the empowerment of women. A man can choose to put on or leave off a condom but a woman has to ask him to do so. This involves a degree of control which some women do not have. A woman may indeed not be a woman at all but a young and inexperienced girl who may not feel able to ask (Holland *et al,* 1990). Different social norms may mean that if she carries condoms she will be thought of as 'easy' or 'loose' and be called a whore or slag. Women are raped or sexually abused and have no power whatsoever to stop the man. They may be economically or emotionally dependent or they may be subject to violence and sex is part of the return that the partner demands. Heterosexual men do not in the main think they are at risk from HIV, and culturally in this country they associate their sexuality with vaginal penetration. They are also conditioned to consider a condom as a reducer of sensation. Society as a whole needs to face these issues. Men need to understand the risks and women need to be enabled to become more assertive and be able to say what they want from sex. No one should die of ignorance or embarrassment. Sex should be fun and sex should be safe.

References

Aboulker, J.P., Swart, A.M. (1993). 'Preliminary analysis of the Concorde trial'. *Lancet* 341, pp. 889-90

Achterberg, J. (1990). *Woman As Healer.* Boston:Shambhala Publications.

AIDS and HIV-1 infection in the United Kingdom (1994). Monthly Report. *Communicable Disease Report* Vol 4, No 15,. 15 April 1994.

Annon, J.S. (1976). 'The PLISTT model: A proposed conceptual scheme for the behavioural treatment of sexual problems. *Journal of Sex Education Therapists* 2, pp.1-15

Archer, J. and Lloyd, B. (1987). *Sex and Gender.* Cambridge: Cambridge University Press.

Ardener, E. (1975). 'Belief and the problem of women'. In: Ardener, S. (Ed). *Perceiving Women 1-17.* London: Dent.

Ardener, S. (1978). *Defining Females : The Nature of Women in Society.* London: Croom Helm

Aries, P. (1985). *Western Sexuality* Oxford: Basil Blackwell.

Avery, M.D. and Burket, B.A. (1986). 'Effect of perineal massage on the incidence of episiotomy and perineal laceration in a nurse-mid-wifery service'. *Journal of Nurse Midwifery* 31, pp. 128-34.

Bailey, V.R. (1989). 'Sexuality - before and after birth'. *Midwives Chronicle & Nursing Notes* Jan, pp. 24-26.

Baker, S. (1980). 'Biological Influences on Human Sex and Gender'. *Signs* 6, pp.80-96.

Ballantyne, A. (1988). 'Doctors forced AIDS virus women to have abortions'. *Guardian* 17th August.

Bancroft J., Myerscough, P. and Schmidt, G. (1983). *Human sexuality and its Problems.* Edinburgh: Churchill livingstone

Bancroft, J., Myerscough, P. and Schmidt, G. (1989). *Human Sexuality and its Problems.* Edinburgh: Churchill Livingstone.

Barnes, J. (1987).*Early Greek Philosophy.* Harmondsworth: Penguin.

Bayer, R. (1981). *Homosexuality and American Psychiatry: The Politics of Diagnosis.* New York: Basic Books.

Behrman, S.J., Kistner, R.W. and Patton, G.W. (1988). *Progress in Infertility.* 3rd Edition. Boston. Little Brown and Co. Ltd.

Berer, M. and Ray, S. (1993). *Women and the HIV/AIDS.* London: Pandora Press.

Bergstrom, L., Roberts, J., Skillman, L. and Seidel, J. (1992). '"You'll feel me touching you sweetie": Vaginal examinations during the second stage of labour'. *Birth* ,March, (1), pp. 10-25.

Berne, E. (1968). *Games People Play* . Harmondsworth: Penguin.

Bewley, C.A. and Gibbs, A. (1991).'Violence in pregnancy'. *Midwifery,* September, (7).pp. 107-12.

Bhaktivedanta Swami Prabhupada AC (1982). *Srimad Bhagavatam. First canto-Part One.* Bath. Pitman Press.

Bohn, D.K. (1990). 'Domestic violence and pregnancy'. *Journal of Nurse Midwifery,* Vol 35, No 2, pp. 86-98.

Brake, M. (Ed). (1982).*Human Sexual Relations.* Harmondsworth: Penguin.

Burns, R.B. (1991). *Essential Psychology.* 2nd Edition. Oxford. Aldern Press.

Byrne, M.A. *et al* (1989). 'The common occurrence of HPV infection and intraepithelial neoplasia in women infected by HIV'. *AIDS* 3,.pp 379-82.

Caplan, P. (1991).*The Cultural Construction of Sexuality.* Suffolk.:Chaucer Press..

Caplan, C. (1992). *The Cultural Construction of Sexuality* New York. Routledge.

Carpenter, C.C.J. (1991). 'HIV infection in north American women: experience with 200 cases and a review of the literature'. *Medicine* 70(5), pp. 307-25.

Chalmers, I., Enkin, M. and Kierse, M.J.N.C. (1989). *Effective Care in Pregnancy and Childbirth.* Oxford: Oxford Universsity Press.

Chodorov, N. (1978).*The Reproduction of Mothering. Psychoanalysis and the Sociology of Gender.* Berkeley: University of California Press.

Close, S. (1984).*Sex During Pregnancy and After Childbirth.* Northamptonshire: Thorson's Publishers Ltd.

Comfort, A. (1987). *More Joy: A Lovemaking Companion to the Joy of Sex.* New York: Crown Publishers.

Cooper, G. and Davidson, M. (1992). *High Pressure: Working Lives of Women Managers.* London: Fontana.

Corea, G. (1992). 'The new reproductive technology: problem or solution? In: Strickler, J. (Ed). *Sociology of Health and Illness,* Vol 14, No1, pp113-32

Courtois, C.A. (1988). *Healing the Incest wound: Adult survivors in therapy* New York. W.W. Norton.

Coward, R. (1984). *Female Desire. Women's Sexuality.* London: Paladin.

Cowling, A.J., Stanworth, M.J.K., Bennett, R.D., Curran, J. and Lyons, P. (1988). *Behavioural Sciences for Managers.* London: Edward Arnold.

Culp, R.E. and Osofsky, H.J. (1989). 'Effects of caesarian section on parental depression, marital adjustment and mother-infant interaction'. *Birth,* June, 16(2),.pp 53-57.

Dannecker, M. (1981).*Theories of Homosexuality.* London. Gay Men's Press.

Darling, C.A. and Davidson, J.K. (1986). 'Enhancing relationships: understanding the feminine mystique of pretending orgasm'. *Journal of Sex and Marital Therapy* 12, No 3, pp.182-96.

De Beauvoir, S. (1988). *The Second Sex.* 3rd edn. London: Jonathan Cape.

Diamond, M., Diamond, A.L. and Mast, M. (1972). 'Visual sensitivity and sexual arousal during the menstrual period'. *Journal of Nervous and Mental Diseases* 155, pp. 170-76.

Dickinson, R.L. and Beam, L. (1932). *A Thousand Marriages.* London: Bailliere, Tindall and Cox.

Donald, I. (1969). 'On launching a new diagnostic science'. *American Journal of Obstetrics and Gynaecology,* March 1, pp. 299-309.

Douglas, M. (1975). *Implicit Meanings: Essays in Anthropology.* London: Routledge.

Douglas, M. (1991). *Purity and Danger: An Analysis of the Concepts of Pollution and Taboo.* London: Routledge.

Draucker, C.B. (1992). *Counselling Survivors of Child Sexual Abuse.* London: Sage Publications Ltd.

Dube, L., Leacock,.E. and Ardener, S. (1986). *Visibility and Power.* Delhi: Oxford University Press.

Duby, G. (1978). *Medievel Marriage.* Baltimore and London: John Hopkins Press.

Dunham, C., Myers, F., Barnden, N., McDougall, A., Kelly, A.L. and Aria, B. (1991). *Mamatoto. A Celebration of Birth.* London: Virago Press.

Ellis Havelock H (1894). *Man and Woman.* London: Walter Scott.

Erhardt, A.A., Ince, S.E. and Mayer-Bahlberg, H.F.L. (1981). 'Career aspirations and gender role development in young girls'. *Archives of Sexual Behaviour.* New York: Wiley.

Erikson, E.H. (1963). *Childhood and Society.* New York: Norton.

European Collaborative Study (1992). 'Risk factors for mother to child transmission of HIV-1'. *Lancet,* 339, pp. 1007-12.

Forbes, T.R. (1966). *The Midwife and the Witch.* London:New Haven.

Flandrin, J. L. (1985). 'Sex in married life in the early middle ages: The Church's teaching and behavioural reality'. In:Aries, P. (Ed). *Western Sexuality.* Oxford: Basil Blackwell.

Flint, C. (1986). *Sensitive Midwifery* Guildford: Heinemann.

Foucault, M. (1973). *The Birth of the Clinic: An Archaeology of Medical Perception.* New York: Pantheon Books.

Foucault, M. (1978). *The History of Sexuality.* Vols I,II,III. London, New York: Penguin.

Foucault, M. (1979). *The History of Sexuality.* Vol 1,2,3. Translater: Hurley, R.. London.: Allen Lane.

Freud, S. (1905). *Three Essays on the Theory of Sexuality.* Vol 7. Standard Edition 1953. London: Hogarth Press.

Freud, S. (1913). 'Totem and taboo'. In: *The Complete Bibliography of Freud's Writings.* New York (1952).Standard Edition 13.1.

Freud, S. (1933). Lecture XX 'The sexual life of man'. In: *Introductory Lectures on Psycho Analysis* (1971).London: Allen and Unwin.

Freud, S. (1962). *Three Essays on the Theory of Sexuality.* Translated by James Strachey. London: Hogarth Press.

Freud, S. (1977). 'On the universal tendency to debasement in the sphere of love'. In: *Freud On Sexuality*. Harmondsworth:Penguin.

Freud, S. (1986). 'Infantile sexuality'. In: *Freud on Sexuality*. Harmondsworth: Penguin.

Freud, S. (1986). *Freud on Sexuality*. Harmondsworth: Penguin.

Froland, S.S. *et al* (1988). 'HIV infection in a Norwegian family before 1970'. *Lancet*, Vol. I, June, Part 8598, pp. 1344-45.

Fuerstein, G. (1990).*Yoga. The Technology of Ecstasy*. Chatham: Mackays.

Furniss, T. (1991).*The Multi Professional Handbook of Child Sexual Abuse; Integrated Management, Therapy and Legal Intervention*. London: Routledge.

Gagnon, J.H. and Simon, W. (1973).*Sexual Conduct*. Chicago: Aldine.

Garai, J.E. and Scheinfeld, A. (1968).'Sex differences in mental and behavioural traits'. *Genetic Psychology Monographs* 77, pp.169-299.

Ghandi, M.K .(1927). *An Autobiography or the Story of my Experiences with Truth*. Ahmedabad: Navajivan Publishing House.

Gillespie, J.G. (1993).'Child sexual abuse 2: techniques for helping adult survivors'. *British Journal of Nursing* Vol 2, No 6, p. 313-15.

Grant, L.J .(1992). 'Efffects of child sexual abuse: issues for obstetric caregivers'. *Birth* 19, 4, Dec, pp. 220-21.

Greer, G. (1969).*The Female Eunuch*. Suffolk: Richard Clay Ltd. and London: Stanley Paul.

Greer, G. (1970).'The politics of female sexuality' In: *The Mad Woman's Underclothes (1986)*. London: Picador.

Haeberle, E.J. (1983).*The Sex Atlas*. London: Sheldon Press.

Havelock Ellis (1959). *Psychology of Sex*. London: Cox and Wyman Ltd.

Hesford, A. and Bhanji, S. (1986). Sexual Dysfunction in Women. *Nursing Times*, April, pp. 49-51.

Hiberman, E. (1990). 'Overview. The wife-beater's wife reconsidered'. *American Journal of Psychiatry* 137, pp.1336-47.

Hirschfield, M. (1953).*Sex in Human Relations*. London: John Lane.

Hite, S. (1976).*The Hite Report*. New York: McMillan

Hite, S. (1984).*The Hite Report on Male Sexuality*. New York: Alfred A Knopf.

Hite, S. (1991).*The Hite Report on Love, Passion and Emotional Violence*. London:. McDonald and Co.

HMSO (1952 to 1990).*Confidential Enquiries in to the Cause of Maternal Deaths in England and Wales*. London: HMSO.

Hogan, R. (1980).'Human sexuality: A nursing perspective'. In: Webb,C. (Ed). *Sexuality, Nursing and Health*. London: J. Wiley & Sons.

Holland, J. *et al* (1990). 'I nearly died of embarrassment'. *Women Risk AIDS Project*. London: The Tufnell Press.

Holmes, K.K., Mardh, P.A., Sparling, P.E., Weisner, P.J., Cates, W., Lemon, S.M. and Stamm, W.E. (1990). *Sexually Transmitted Diseases*. 2nd Edition. New York: McGraw Hill.

Horney K. (1924). 'On the genesis of the castration complex in women'. *International Journal of Psychoanalysis*. 5, pp.50-65.

Hubbard, R. (1985). 'Prenatal diagnosis and eugenic ideology'. *Women's Studies International Forum* 8, 6, pp 567-76.

Ingrey, J. (1993). 'Water birth. A press release'. *Midwifery Matters* 59; p.6.

Jackson, M. (1991). 'Facts of life or the eroticization of women's oppression? Sexology and the social construction of heterosexuality'. In: Caplan, P. (Ed). *The Cultural Construction of Sexuality*. New York: Routledge.

Jacobus, M. (1990). *Body Politics - Women and the Discourse of Science*. London: Routledge.

Jeffrey, P., Jeffrey, R. and Lyon, A. (1989). *Labour Pains and Labour Power*. London: Zed Books.

Kelly, J. (1988). 'Genital herpes during pregnancy'. *British Mediacal Journal*, Vol 297, No 6657, November, pp. 1146-47.

Kenny, J.A. (1976).'Sexual attitudes and behaviour patterns during and following pregnancy'. *Archives of Sexual Behaviour* 5, pp.539-51.

Kessler, S.J. and McKenna, W. (1978).*Gender, an Ethnomethodological Approach*. New York: Wiley.

Kessler, S.J .and McKenna, W. (1987).*Gender An Methodological Approach*. New York: Wiley.

Kinsey, A.C., Pomeroy, W.B., Martin, C.E. and Gebhard, P.H. (1953).*Sexual Behaviour in the Human Female*. Philadelphia. W.B. Saunders Co.

Kinsey Institute (1958).*Pregnancy, Birth and Abortion*. Philiadelphia: W B Saunders and Co.

Kinsey Institute (1965).*Sex Offenders: An Analysis of Types*. London: Thomas Nelson.

Kinsey, S. (1991).*The Kinsey Institute New Report on Sex*. London: Penguin.

Kirkham, M. (1989). 'Midwives and information giving during labour'. In: Robinson, S and Thomson, A.M. (Eds). *Midwives, Research and Childbirth*, Vol 1. London: Chapman and Hall.

Kitzinger, S. (1983).*Woman's Experience of Sex*. London: Dorling Kindersley.

Kitzinger, C. (1987).*The Social Construction of Lesbianism*. London.: Sage Publications.

Kitzinger, S. (1991). *Homebirth and Other Alternatives to Hospital*. London: Dorling Kindersley.

Kitzinger, J. V. (1992). 'Counteracting, not re-enacting, the violation of women's bodies: the challenge for perinatal caregivers'. *Birth* 19, 4, Dec, pp. 219-20.

Kohlberg, L. and Ullian, D. (1974). 'Stages in the development of psychosexual concepts and attitudes'. In: Maccoby, E. (Ed). *The Development of Sex Differences*. Stanford: Stanford University Press.

Kramer, L. (1990). *Reports from the Holocaust. The Making of an AIDS Survivor*. Harmondsworth: Penguin.

Kromemeyer, R. (1980). *Overcoming Homosexuality*. New York: Macmillan.

Lacan, J. (1977). *Ecrits: A Selection*. London: Tavistock.

Levi-Strauss, C. (1969). *The Elementary Structures of Kinship*. Boston: Beacon Press.

Lewis, M. (1975). 'Early sex differences in the human: studies of socioemotional development'. *Archives of Sexual Behaviour* 4, pp.329-35.

Lewis, I.M. (1976). *Social Anthropology in Perspective* Cambridge: Cambridge University Press.

Litvinoff, S. (1992). *The Relate Guide to Sex in Loving Relationships*. London: Vermilion.

Maseide, P. (1991). 'Possibly abusive, often benign, and always necessary. On power and domination in medical practice'. *Sociology of Health and Illness*. Vol 13, No 4, .

Masters, W.H. and Johnson, V.E. (1966). *Human Sexual Response* Boston. Little, Brown and Co.

McKenna, H.P. (1991). 'The developments and trends in relation to men practising midwifery: A review of the literature'. *Journal of Advanced Nursing* 16, pp.480-89.

McNamara, R.J. (1989). *Towards Balance*. Maine: Samuel Weiser.

Mead, M. (1974). *Los Angeles Times*., 5 February, part 4. p.6. In: Oakley, A (1990). *The Captured Womb: A History of the Medical Care of Pregnant Women* Oxford: Basil Blackwell.

Melzack, R. and Wall, P.D. (1965). 'Pain mechanisms: A new theory'. *Science,* 150, p.971.

MENCAP, 123 Golden Lane, London. EC1.

Mercey, D., Bewley, S. and Brocklehurst, P. (1993). *A Guide to HIV Infection and Childbearing*. Horsham: Avert.

Merson, M. (1990). *Report of the Meeting on Research Priorities Relating to Women and HIV/AIDS*. World Health Organisation Global Programme on AIDS. November 19/20 (3).

Merton, R.K. (1970). 'The role set: problems in sociological theory'. In: Worsley, P. (Ed). *Modern Sociology: Introductory Readings*. London: Penguin.

MIND, 22 Harley St, London, W1N 2ED.

Mitchell, J. (1974). *Psychoanalysis and Feminism*. London: Allen Lane.

Money, J. (1965). 'Psychosexual differentiation'. In: *Sex Research, New Developments*. New York: Wiley.

Money, J. and Erhadt, A.A. (1972). *Man and Woman, Boy and Girl*. Baltimore: John Hopkins University Press.

Money, J., Hampson, J.L. and Hampson, J.G. (1955). 'An examination of some basic sexual concepts: the evidence of human hermaphroditism'. *Bulletins of John Hopkins Hospital* 97, pp.301-19.

Moore, J. (1982). 'A man's job?' *Nursing Times* 78(10), p.398.

Moore, H.J. (1988).*Feminism and Anthropology*. Cambridge. Polity Press.

Moss, H.A. (1970). 'Sex, age and state as determinants of mother- infant interaction'. In: Danziger, K. (Ed). *Readings in Child Socialisation*. Oxford: Pergamon Press

Mynaugh, P.A. (1991). 'A randomised study of two methods of teaching perineal massage: effect on practice rates, episiotomy rates, and lacerations'. *Birth*, 18/3, pp 153-59.

Najman,,J.M. *et al* (1991).'The mental health of women six months after they give birth to an unwanted baby: A longitudinal study'. *Social Science & Medicine*, Vol. 32, Part 3, pp.241-47.

Nass, G.D. and Fisher, M.P. (1988).*Sexuality Today*. Boston: Jones and Bartlett Publishers.

Nelson,A.M. *et al* (1991). 'Increased rates of cervical dysplasia associated with clinical and immunological evidence of immunodeficiency'. *6th International Conference on AIDS in Africa*, Dakar 16-19 December 1991, Abstract No W.A. 209

New Jersey Women and AIDS Network (1990). *Me first, Medical Manifestations of HIV in Women* New Brunswick: New Brunswick Press.

Newell, M.L. and Peckham,C. (1993). 'Risk factors for vertical transmission of HIV-1 and early markers of HIV-1 infection in children'. *AIDS* 7, (Suppl 1).S91-S97.

Newton, N., Peeler, D. and Newton, M. (1968). 'Effect of disturbance in labour'. *American Journal of Obstetrics and Gynaecology* 90, p.118.

Oakley, A. (1990).*The Captured Womb: A History of the Medical Care of Pregnant Women*. Oxford: Basil Blackwell Ltd.

Oliver, M. (1990).*The Politics of Disablement*. Basingstoke:Macmillan.

Ortner, S.B. (1973).'On key symbols'. *American Anthroplogist* 75, pp. 1338-46.

Ortner, S.B. (1974). 'Is female to male as nature is to culture?' In: Rosaldo, M. and Lamphere, L. (Eds).*Woman, Culture and Society* 67-68. Stanford: Stanford University Press.

Ortner, S.B. and Whitehead, H. (1981). *Sexual Meanings. The Cultural Construction of Gender*. Cambridge: Cambridge University Press.

Parsons, T. (1967). *Sociological Theory and Modern Society*. New York: Free Press.

Piaget, J. (1952).*The Origins of Intelligence in Children*. New York: Internatinal Universities Press.

Poff, D. (1987). 'Content, intent and consequences: life production and reproductive technology'. *Atlantis,* Vol 13, pp.111-13.

Pryce, A. (1991). 'Expressing sexuality'. *Nursing*. Vol 4, No 4, pp. 15-16.

Quadagno, D.M., Briscoe, R. and Quadagno, J.S. (1977). 'Effect of prenatal gonadal hormones on selected nonsexual behaviour patterns: A critical assessment of the human and non human literature'. *Psychological Bulletin* 84, pp.62-80.

Rattray Taylor, G. (1953).*Sex in History*. London: Thames and Hudson.

Raymond, J.G. (1979). *The Transsexual Empire*. Boston: Beacon Press.

Reeler, A.V. (1990). 'Injections: A fatal attraction?' *Social Science and Medicine* 31(10),.pp 1119-25.

Reinich, J.M. and Beasley, R. (1990). *The New Kinsey Report on Sex*. London: Penguin.

Richards, L.B. (1992). 'The perpetuation of fear and cesarean'. *Midwifery Today* Autumn, No 23, pp. 20-21.

Richardson, D. (1989). *Women and the AIDS Crisis*. London: Pandora.

Robson, K.M. (1982). 'Falling interest'. *Nursing Mirror* June 16, pp. 42-45.

Roper, N., Logan, W. and Tierney, A. (1985). *The Elements of Nursing*. 2nd Edition. Edinburgh: Churchill Livingstone.

Rose, A. (1992). 'Effects of sexual abuse on childbirth: one woman's story'. *Birth* 19, 4 December, pp. 214-18.

Ross, C. (1986). 'Let it rip? The healing of the perineum following spontaneous vaginal delivery'. *Research and the Midwife Conference Proceedings, Glasgow*. Dept. of Nursing Studies, Manchester University.

Rubin, G.S. (1993). 'Thinking sex'. In: Abelove, H., Barale, M.A. and Halpern, D.M. (1993). *The Lesbian and Gay Studies Reader*. New York: Routledge.

Savage, J. (1987). *Nurses, Gender and Sexuality*. London: Heinneman.

Shainess, N. (1984). *Sweet Suffering: Woman as Victim*. New York: Bobs Merrill.

Shakespeare, W. (1989). *As You Like It,* Act II, Scene 7. New York: Routledge.

Sherif, M. (1936). *The Psychology of Social Norms*. London: Harper.

Simkin, P. (1992). 'Ovecoming the legacy of child sexual abuse: The role of caregivers and childbirth educators'. *Birth* 19, 4, Dec, pp 224-25.

Sleep, J. and Grant, A. (1987). 'Pelvic floor exercises in postnatal care'. *Midwifery*, 3 (4), pp. 158-64.

Sleep, J. and Grant, A. (1989). 'Perineal pain and discomfort'. In: Enkin, M., Kierse, M. and Chalmers, I. (Eds). *Effective Care in Pregnancy and Childbirth*. Oxford: Oxford University Press.

Speak, M. and Aitken-Swan, J. (1982). *Male midwives: A Report of Two Studies*. London: HMSO.

SPOD (Sexual and Personal Relations of the Disabled), 286 Camden Rd, London,. N7 OBJ.

Stanworth, M. (1987). *Reproductive Technologies: Gender, Motherhood and Medicine*. Cambridge: Polity Press.

Stockard, J. and Johnson, M. (1979). 'The social origins of male dominance'. *Sex Roles* 5, pp.199-218.

Stoller, R. (1968). *Sex and Gender*. London: Hogarth.

Stopes, M. and Chance, A. (1952). In: Stone, H. and Sone, A. (Eds). *A Marriage Manual*. London: Gollancz.

Stanworth, M. (1988). *Reproductive Technologies: Gender, Motherhood and Medicine*. Cambridge: Basil Blackwell Ltd.

Swain, J., Finkelstein, V., French, S. and Oliver, M. (1993). *Disabling Barriers - Enabling Environments*. London: Sage Publications.

Thomas, K. (1971). *Religion and the Decline of Magic* London: Penguin Books.

Tisdall, S. (1993). 'Lesbian loses custody of toddler to her disapproving mother'. *The Guardian Newspaper,* 9 September, p.11.

Tozzi, A. E. *et al* (1990). 'Does breastfeeding delay progression to AIDS in HIV infected children?' *AIDS* 4,.pp. 1293-94.

Turner, V. (1974).*Dramas, Fields and Metaphors.* Cornell: Cornell university Press.

Van Gennep, A. (1960).*The Rites of Passage.* Chicago: University of Chicago Press.

Vincent, S. (1993). 'Lost boys'. *The Guardian Newspaper,* 16 October, p. 4.

Walton, I. (1993). 'Women labour, men time: an ethnographic study of the labour ward'. Unpublished MSc Dissertation. Keele University.

Warnock, M. (1984).*A Question of Life: The Warnock Report on Human Fertilisation and Embryology* London: HMSO.

Watson, C. (1991). 'Sexual roles in nursing'. *Nursing,* Vol 4, No 4, pp. 13-16.

Weale, S. (1993). 'Lesbian couple win three year struggle to foster young children but victory "provides no charter"'. *The Guardian,* 21 April, p 5.

Weeks, G. (1991).*Sexuality,* Suffolk: Richard Clay Ltd.

Weeks, J. (1983). *Sex, Politics and Society. The regulation of Sexuality since 1800.* London and New York: Longman.

White, D. and Wollett, A. (1981). 'The family at birth'. Paper presented at the British Psychological Society, London Conference, December 1981.

WHO/UNICEF consultation on HIV transmission and Breast feeding. Consensus statement and press release, Geneva 4 May 1992.

Wittig, M. (1993). 'One is not born a woman'. In: Abelove, H. *et al.* (Eds). *The Lesbian and Gay Studies Reader.* New York: Routledge.

Wolf, D.G. (1980). *The Lesbian Community.* Berkeley: University of California Press.

Worwood, V.A. (1992).*The Fragrant Pharmacy. A complete Guide to Aromatherapy and Essential Oils.* London: Bantam Books.

Wright, A. (1994).'Perineal pain after childbirth'. *Midwives Chronicle and Nursing Notes,* Vol 107, No 1, 272, pp. 22-23.

Ziegler, J., Cooper, D. *et al.* (1985). 'Postnatal transmission of AIDS associated retrovirus from mother to infant'. *Lancet,* Vol. II, pp. 896-98.

* All Biblical References are taken from The Revised Standard Edition of the Holy Bible.

The Book of Common Prayer and Administration of the Sacraments and Other Rites and Ceremonies of the Church According To the Use of The Church of England (1662).1968 edition. London: Cambridge University Press.

The Alternative Service Book (1980.).Margate: Eyre and Spottiswoode Ltd.

Index

clitoridectomy 132
clitoris 13, 29, 30, 39, 40, 44, 46, 47, 48, 49, 55, 80, 93, 101, 103
Close 79
coitus 32, 40, 43, 49, 50, 52, 54, 57, 76, 81, 88
coitus interruptus 8
colostomy 70
colporrhaphy 71
Comfort 49
condoms 56, 155
congenital abnormalities 147, 153
contraception 34, 56, 66, 107, 111, 114
contraceptive 60, 65, 77, 150
Corea 26
coronary 70
corpus luteum 18, 57
Courtois 120
Cowling 108
Cowper's glands 42, 44, 45
Cucchiari 15
cunnilingus 49, 80, 154
cytomegalovirus 147, 153

D

De Beauvoir, Simone 13, 26, 31, 37, 121, 130
defloration 11
diabetes 69, 79, 81
Diamond 46
Dickinson and Beam 13
disability 63, 64, 65, 68, 72
doctor 15, 70, 71, 81, 82, 93, 94, 117, 119, 121, 136
Donald 122
Douglas 12, 21, 98
Draucker 91, 119
Dunham 90
dyspareunia 71, 82, 93, 94, 102

E

Earth Mother Goddess 10, 132
ego 27, 28, 62
Electra 30, 31
Ellis
  Havelock 13, 27, 32
emphysema 69
enema 93, 123
epididymis 42, 43
episiotomy 47, 93, 94, 95, 101, 102, 150
Equal Opportunities Legislation 22
erection 45, 47, 52, 53, 59, 61, 68, 77, 139
Erhardt 19
Erhardt, Ince and Mayer-Bahlberg 19
Erikson 53, 56

F

Factory Acts 25
fallopian tubes 17, 40, 41, 43, 57, 72, 73, 84
fellatio 49, 80, 154
fertility control 13
Flandrin, Jean-Louis 7
Flint 88, 93
follicle stimulating hormone 18, 54, 57
Forbes 10
forceps deliveries 94
Foucault 4, 37, 64, 100
Freud 5, 12, 27, 28, 29, 30, 31, 33, 46, 52, 58, 131, 134
frigidity 13, 32, 33, 105
Fuerstein 62
Furniss 129